UPGRADE Your Breath
UPGRADE Your Health

By Logan Christopher
www.LegendaryStrength.com

DISCLAIMER

The exercises and training information contained within this book may be too strenuous or dangerous for some people, and the reader should consult with a physician before engaging in them. The health advice contained within this book is for educational purposes only and is not intended for medical purposes.

The author and publisher of this book are not responsible in any manner whatsoever for the use, misuse or dis-use of the information presented here.

All images, unless otherwise noted, are from my private collection. They are reproduced here under the professional practice of fair use for the purposes of historical discussion and scholarly interpretation. All characters and images remain the property of their respective copyright holders.

Published by:

Legendary Strength LLC

Santa Cruz, California

www.LegendaryStrength.com

Table of Contents

Introduction to the Upgrade Your Health Series

Upgrade Your Health is all about taking where you're currently at with one aspect of your health and bringing it up to a higher level. It's not a matter of doing it wrong, or doing it right. While some things are clearly bad or clearly good, this isn't a game of black and white. Instead there are many shades of grey. There is lots of room for better or worse. Sometimes there will be a best and worst, but when you look at that, the answer can be malleable and changing over time, especially when it comes to you as an individual.

Ideally, you'd want to be at the top end of the spectrum, but for a variety of reasons you may not be able to get there immediately. If you can, great, make that leap. But even if you can just climb one rung up the ladder, that step will improve your health. Then after some time you can make the next step, and so on, until you reach the top.

In some cases, there may not always be a clear answer on what is the best. And since everyone is individual you have to experiment and find what works best for you and your lifestyle.

Either way, by taking the incremental approach, or the big leap to betterment, you can work towards the goal of "Radiant Health". I first heard of this Daoist idea from one of my teachers, Ron Teeguarden. The idea behind this is that you reach a place of "health beyond danger". That means a place where sickness and disease cannot affect you. It's a good place to be at! So how do you get there? By upgrading all the different areas of health.

Unfortunately, it's not as simple as take this pill, or eat this, not that. There's much more to health than that. And I would argue that the majority of people are spending too much time on the wrong things. For instance, what you eat, while important, isn't the whole picture. The truth is if you upgrade every other area of health then what you eat won't be that important. And doing so can be both fun and easy to do. It can become a challenging exploration that gives you bountiful rewards.

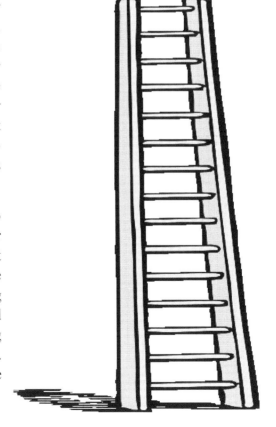

Furthermore, by upgrading your health you can also upgrade your performance. By having all of your bodily systems working for you, rather than against you, you'll find that gaining strength, skill and the body you desire becomes much easier to do. By doing all the things that best support your health you'll find your body will automatically move towards looking its best. This is because form follows function. Optimize the function of your systems and "the system" will look and work great.

Your energy will improve. So, will your cognition and your ability to be productive and hit any goal you desire. Great health is one thing many successful people have in common.

Most of what we focus on in this series could be called the basics. However, as you'll come to see, there are lots of details that can go into these basics. We'll dive deep into each topic giving you every detail I can give from all of my research and personal experimentation to help you upgrade where you're at.

In my earlier books *101 Simple Steps to Radiant Health* and *101 Advanced Steps to Radiant Health*, I delivered a bunch of tips to upgrade your health. While there may be a collection of tips on a specific topic, it wasn't structured in a way like this series is designed to be. Here you can dive into one topic deeply to bring it to the next level.

Yet looking with this much detail can often be overwhelming. But by diving into this detailed view then zooming back out to the bigger picture we can learn many things that we can then implement into our lives. As always, this guide ends with a condensed action plan of what to do to really upgrade this area of your health. So, without further ado…

The Importance of Breathing

"Breathing exercises alone, if done right, will make many a weak man strong and many a sick man well." - Martin 'Farmer' Burns

That quote from one of the greatest wrestlers of all time was instrumental in my early focus on breathwork and how it could be used to increase my health and strength. Recent research backs up Burns' claim.

In the Framingham Heart Study[1], started in 1948, with 5000 subjects from Framingham, Massachusetts an important correlation was found. Every other year involved a physical examination of all participants involving a variety of tests and measurements. What was found was that the vital capacity of the lungs had a high correlation to heart disease. One of the doctors involved in the study, William B. Kannel of the Boston School of Medicine said "Long before a person becomes terminally ill, vital capacity can predict lifespan."

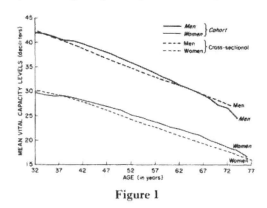

Figure 1

Average age trends in vital capacity levels for cross-sectional and cohort data: Framingham Study, exams 1-10.

1

Other studies have examined this as well, finding how reduced respiratory function correlates with suppressed immune function as well. In fact, it may be one of the best indicators, besides age, to predict illness and death.

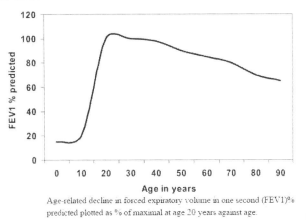

Age-related decline in forced expiratory volume in one second (FEV1)% predicted plotted as % of maximal at age 20 years against age.

2

Thus, we might extrapolate that increasing your lung power is one of the best anti-aging practices you could possibly do. It is free to do. No gym memberships, equipment or buying food or supplements is required. Add that to the fact that it is super simple to get started and it seems that our health journey ought to begin with breathing. Everything else we do comes after that. It is the foundation.

And its practice has gone far back in time. Greek and Roman physicians recommended daily breathing exercises and holding the breath, what they called *"Cohibitio Spiritus"* for their curative powers.

Yet most of our thoughts about health are focused on nutrition. Then there are the lifestyle factors like sleep and exercise. Seldom do we pay much attention to breath.

This probably occurs because each of us breathes automatically and thus it doesn't seem like a big deal. "I don't need to be taught how to breathe," they say, "I know how to do it already." And while that is true, anyone interested in health spends time learning how to eat better, sleep better and move better. Books, seminars and coaching all exist around those subjects.

Yet the breath may be the most important. The simple fact is that you can go over a month without food, weeks without sleep and maybe over a week without water. But even the most advanced practitioners of holding the breath can't go more than a half hour without air. (The record at the time of this writing is 22 minutes 22 seconds by Tom Sietas, a German freediver. This was done by first hyperventilating with oxygen.) And the average person wouldn't even last three minutes, though by the time you finish this guide and put it into practice you'll be able to far exceed that.

Here's some interesting stats that might help you to further understand the value of breathwork. Each day the average person breathes in 360 cubic feet, or 2000 gallons of air. This air had a total weight of 25 lbs. That is three times as much as the total weight of food and liquids taken in by the average person each day.

Of course, it is not just about the amount of air you breathe. A big part is the way in which you do it. We will be covering a wide variety of different kinds of breathing drills that are done for different purposes throughout this book. Several of these purposes include breathing for health, lung capacity, relaxation, strength, endurance, flexibility and to move energy as well as to bridge the gap between the conscious and subconscious. Even with all that, different types of breathing are only one part of the breathing equation.

Many people will tell you there is a right way and a wrong way to breathe. They tend to stick to a single way and say that's the best method of breathing. While there are certainly some basic principles, the reason you can breathe in so many different ways, means that there are different uses. Any one drill is not necessarily better than another.

I like to think of breathing as a movement. As a movement, it's good the more variety you can do. Is it good to do weighted squats or bodyweight squats? While many people would argue one may be better than other, the simple answer is that both are good and bring about some similar as well as different benefits. Breathing is similar. Why not just work to use your breathing in a wide variety of ways?

That's exactly what we'll be doing, covering a wide variety of drills so you can find what works best for you. In fact, more types of breathing are covered here than in any other resource on the subject that I've ever seen. An alternate name for this book could be the 'Encyclopedia of Breathing Exercises'.

The last part, that may be just as important, is the quality of the air that you breathe. The air in our polluted cities, and how we recycle air in our buildings, is not the best for our health. Thus, a section of this manual will cover what you can do to upgrade your environment, even if you are trapped indoors. We'll finish off with some herbal remedies that can assist in the health of your lungs and respiratory tract.

Ultimately, when you gain greater control of your breathing you can use it for a wide variety of functions. You'll also improve your health through better functioning lungs and with better air quality. All of these things are the end result of *Upgrade Your Breath*.

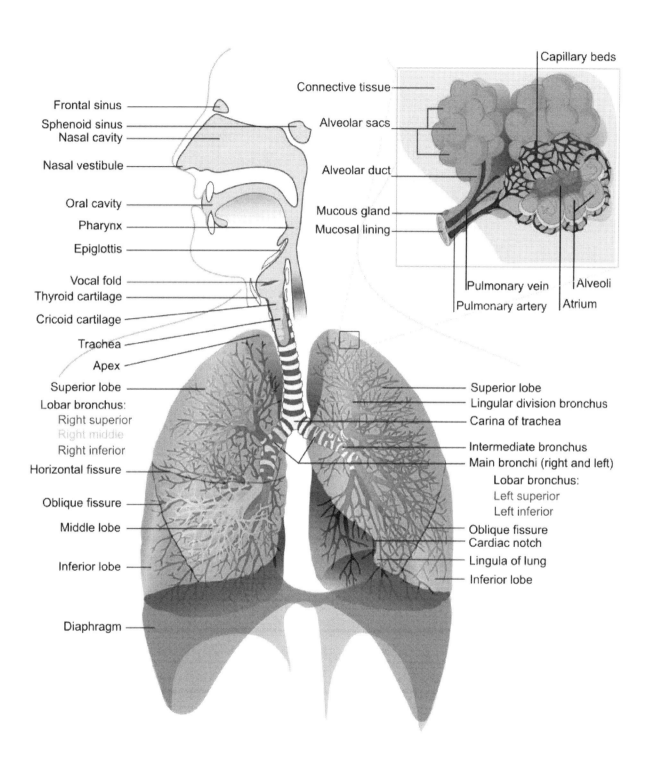

Frontal sinus
Sphenoid sinus
Nasal cavity
Nasal vestibule
Oral cavity
Pharynx
Epiglottis
Vocal fold
Thyroid cartilage
Cricoid cartilage
Trachea
Apex
Superior lobe
Lobar bronchus:
  Right superior
  Right middle
  Right inferior
Horizontal fissure
Oblique fissure
Middle lobe
Inferior lobe
Diaphragm

Capillary beds
Connective tissue
Alveolar sacs
Alveolar duct
Mucous gland
Mucosal lining
Pulmonary vein
Pulmonary artery
Alveoli
Atrium

Superior lobe
Lingular division bronchus
Carina of trachea
Intermediate bronchus
Main bronchi (right and left)
Lobar bronchus:
  Left superior
  Left inferior
Oblique fissure
Cardiac notch
Lingula of lung
Inferior lobe

How the Respiratory System Works

"It is a common belief that we breathe with our lungs alone, but in point of fact, the work of breathing is done by the whole body." – Alexander Lower, The Voice of the Body

Before we dive into the different forms of breathing and why to do them it is helpful to have a basic understanding of the anatomy and physiology of the respiratory system, which includes the lungs and much more. Some of these details will become important in later sections so it is good to start here.

The respiratory system is commonly divided into two sections, the upper and lower. The upper respiratory tract includes the nose, mouth, pharynx, larynx and trachea. Air is breathed in through the nose or mouth and then moves through the throat into the lower respiratory tract. It is important to note that a large portion of the lymphatic system is in this area to fight any pathogens. The tonsils and other lymph tissue are part of the immune system.

The picture on the preceding page covers many more of the anatomical terms, most of which aren't important for our purposes here. It also gives a close up view in the upper right hand corner, of the alveoli in the lungs.

The upper respiratory tract is also called the conducting zone. Its function is to purify, humidify and warm the incoming air.

The lower respiratory tract is made up of the bronchial tree, lungs and the alveoli. From the trachea the air then branches into two tubes, the bronchi which feed into each lung. These tubes then further subdivide, branching into more and more bronchioles. Eventually, these end in the alveoli which are small air sacs where the exchange of oxygen, carbon dioxide and water takes place.

Many people think of the lungs as hollow but a better description would be sponge-like. They're only about 10% solid tissue, the rest being filled with air and blood. The heart pumps blood directly to the lungs for the gas exchange and then back to itself to spread oxygenated blood throughout the body.

Another common misconception is that the lungs are in the front of the torso. In actuality, about two thirds of the mass of the lungs are closer to the back than the front.

The lungs are coated in mucosal tissue which helps to keep them moist. Surrounding the lungs is a protective membrane called the pleura or pleural membrane which contains synovial fluid, the same as is in your joints, so that friction doesn't cause damage in its constant contraction and expansion.

The lungs are innervated by the vagus nerve. Both the autonomic and central nervous system are at play in the role of breathing which is why it is both under conscious and unconscious control. It's amazing to think that you're taking roughly 14000-24000 breaths each day!

The Diaphragm

One of the critical pieces of the respiratory system is the diaphragm. This is sometimes also called the thoracic diaphragm, as it is located near the middle or thoracic spine. The diaphragm is a skeletal muscle that separates the heart and lungs from the abdominal cavity.

As a muscle, it is used in expanding the area available to the lungs, by pushing the other organs downward, allowing the lungs to fill with more air. This is why in deep breathing the belly ends up extending, because more room needs to be made. This is often called diaphragmatic breathing as this muscle is being put to use.

Because it is inside of the body, you may not think of it as much as those muscles that you can see, but this is one muscle that is active pretty much all of the time. Its contraction is used in every inhale, while it relaxes in every exhale. And as a muscle it can become stronger, or weaker, depending on use. Of all your muscles is might be one of the most important to focus on developing.

The diaphragm is not the only breathing muscle though. A normal exhale is done through elastic recoil of the lungs and other tissues. But a forced exhale is supported by the intercostals, the muscles lining the ribs, and the abdominal muscles as well.

In short, doing a variety of different types of breathing exercises will help to make sure all these muscles, organs and systems stay healthy. With the human body, it is use it or lose it, and this certainly applies here.

Principles of Breath Work

"Then the LORD God formed man of dust from the ground, and breathed into his nostrils the breath of life; and man became a living being." – Genesis 2:7

Before we get into specific exercises it is important to note the principles behind all of the breath work we will be doing. The following six areas come into play, mixed and matched, in just about everything else covered in this book. If you can understand and use these principles, that is much better than just knowing a bunch of different types of breathing drills. Thus, it will be useful to cover each of them in full here before getting into specific applications.

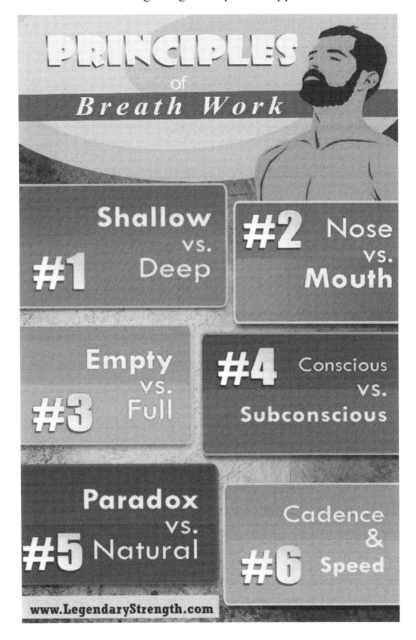

Principle #1 – Shallow vs. Deep Breathing

One of the most important parts of breathing lies in how much of your lungs you're actually using in order to do it. It is often called shallow breathing when not that much air is coming in, and deep breathing when the lungs are more fully used.

Although the term may be confusing, another way to think of shallow breathing is when it is high up in the chest. As such, only the top part of the lungs are being put to use, the air shallowly penetrating into the body. This can often be seen in other people with the chest and even sometimes the shoulders raising up.

One time when I was at a conference, the speaker onstage was telling people to do deep breathing. I was standing in the back of the room and saw this woman in front of me. Her idea of deep breathing was shrugging her shoulders up towards her ears. Unfortunately for her, this is not how you breathe deeply.

It's not just one or the other but varying degrees of shallow or deep. The middle breath may still see the chest expanding but it will also expand the ribs. The deep breath will finally see action in the diaphragm with the belly expanding as well.

It is important to note that different people may naturally favor a more shallow or deep type of breathing. In NLP (neuro-linguistic programming), you can notice the 'visual' person because they are typically shallow breathers. Contrast this to the 'kinesthetic' person who is a much deeper breather, and the 'auditory' person being somewhere in the middle.

That being said, for oxygenation of the tissues, the deeper breathing is what we want and it is a trainable skill. By consciously doing deep breathing drills, many varieties of which will be covered, you'll begin to subconsciously breathe deeper too. The aim is to make it a habit that the body does so without you having to think about it.

To really get a feel for this we turn to a remedial drill. If you've never focused on your breathing in this way before, you may not have the awareness or physical control of your body to do so. This drill can help point you towards what needs to be done.

Lie on your back and place a light object on your stomach. A shoe or a book works just fine. First, we'll start with a shallow breath merely to note the contrast. Breathe into your upper chest and notice that the object and your stomach do not need to move. You can raise your head to look at the object, or keep your hand on it to feel where it is at.

Now this time take a deep breath. Inhale lower into your lungs, which will push the diaphragm, and in turn raise your stomach. Doing so the object will move upwards, and with the exhale, downwards. Do not push your belly out but allow it to move as you breathe deep. Continue breathing like this for ten breaths or so, getting a feel for deep breathing.

The object is there merely as a point of focus so you can see it raise and fall with the proper deep breathing. Once you get the feel of what it takes to move the object through breathing, you can do away with it and deep breathe in any position you desire.

As deep breathing allows more air in, it is going to be a common element in most of the techniques done throughout this guide, but not all of them. Remember that the more you practice it consciously, the more it will become a habit that is handled by the unconscious too. Our goal here is to have unconscious competency in deep breathing. Doing so will bring about various health benefits.

Principle #2 - Nose vs. Mouth

Breathing can be done through either the nose or the mouth. Is one better than the other? The short answer is yes. The long answer is it depends. It is preferable to breathe through the nose, at least when inhaling, though there are exceptions. One of the main reasons is filtration. This doesn't just occur if you have nose hairs, which certainly can help with larger particles, but also in the nasal concha where cilia and mucous can absorb smaller particles and allergens.

Other benefits of nasal breathing include warming and moistening the air on the inhale and reducing the amount of moisture lost on the exhale.

Another more advanced aspect of nasal breathing is that nitric oxide (NO) from the sinuses gets mixed with the air, which enhances oxygenation of the blood. This does not occur when breathing in through the mouth and in one study was shown to deliver 10-18% more oxygen to the arteries and cells[3].

On more of an energetic level, the mouth closed with the tongue resting up against the roof of the mouth is considered a good default position for it. This helps to connect the central and governing vessels as described in Chinese medicine. This will often be recommended with qi gong or meditation practices, such as the microcosmic orbit, to be covered later.

For these reasons, nasal breathing should be your default. If it is not currently, as before with deep breathing, this is a trainable skill that can be built consciously so that it eventually becomes unconscious habit.

Of course, there is a time and a place for mouth breathing. When you push yourself to a certain level physically, you're going to have to switch. The reason for this is simply because the mouth is bigger than the nose. You're able to get more air in and also expel more out by using the mouth compared to the nose. This need only be done when you have pushed yourself to the level where you require more oxygen and need to remove more carbon dioxide from your body.

Yet there are times when you want to focus on nose breathing even when you are doing endurance exercises. And there are times when mouth breathing may be useful besides just in endurance training.

Unfortunately, there are two health issues that can make nasal breathing harder to do. In Weston A. Price's *Nutrition and Physical Degeneration*, what he talks about is not just the tooth decay that happens, but actually the change in the bone structure, both in the mouth and the nasal passages, as a result of eating improper foods (what he called "the white man foods"). This is even worse off today than back in his almost eighty years ago. This isn't actually about your nutrition, but your parents primarily, and in turn their parents and so on.

If you're not familiar with Price's work he studied the native diets of natural living people and found virtually no dental caries or tooth decay, even though the diets often differed wildly. This was in stark contrast to the people of Western culture, or when these indigenous people starting eating industrialized foods. The formation of natural people's faces are also much better, with degradation seeming to narrow breathing passageways. So, while this may be outside of your control, I don't think many people will be deformed so much that nasal breathing won't work for them.

Which brings us to the more common difficulty with nasal breathing that is within your control. If you're always congested, you may not be able to get sufficient air flow. Congestion happens primarily because of a buildup of mucus.

Mucus formation is caused by many foods. It's not bad in and of itself. Recall that the mucous membrane is part of our defense system, as well as keeping things lubricated so our aim is not to get rid of all mucus. But excessive amounts can become stagnant and build up.

The biggest culprit in this is dairy products. Many people are intolerant of these, though not everyone. Of course, any food allergens could possibly contribute to this issue. Personally, refined grains and gluten will cause me to get stuffed up. By cutting down or eliminating these foods you can make your breathing much easier. You can also eat more mucus clearing foods like olive oil, figs, ginger, onion, cayenne, citrus fruits and most greens.

Another option that can help to cleanse the nasal passages is a neti pot, which is a small device that is used to pour salt water or saline solution up one nostril and allow it to drain out the other. I've heard it described as brushing your teeth for your nose. It helps to clear out the junk that can be trapped in there.

Principle #3 - Empty vs. Full

At first thought this may appear to be the same thing as shallow vs. deep breathing, but it is an important distinction. This refers to how much of a breath you are taking rather than where it is located.

Go ahead and try this simple drill right now. Breathe low into your belly but only take a small breath, less so than you would normally take. Exhale. Now breathe again deep into your belly but with a full breath. Let go. Now take a shallow breath, into the chest, but only a small sip of air. Exhale again. Follow that up by taking a full breath starting high up in the chest but keeping it high. Let it out. For this final breath, start a low breath and breathe in fully. Keep breathing in until the chest and even shoulders expand a little bit.

So you can see there is a difference in the location as well as the volume of breath. The word 'deep' can mean both low and high volume, but our distinction here refers to lower, or deeper, into the body. Shallow also can refer to location, only shallowly penetrating into the lungs, or volume, as in not much of it. Once again, our use of it here is for location.

Contrast that to empty and full. Empty obviously would mean no breath at all. It is important to note that you cannot fully empty the lungs. Even when you forcefully exhale there is still residual air left. If you could actually force all the air out, your lungs would be damaged. If we talk about an empty breath, speaking about the inhale, this would be a small amount of air. Unfortunately, this is how most people breathe regularly.

A fun little experiment is to watch a timer for one minute and count how many breaths you do. If you do this yourself you'll be conscious of your breathing and thus are likely to slow it down, however if you had someone watch from the outside and do this you might be surprised as how 'empty' your breathing might be.

The end goal of natural breathing for us here would be both deep and close to full breaths. They shouldn't be completely full as that takes effort to expand your lungs fully, but more volume of air than what most people do.

In this book, we will cover different drills that work to expand both the emptiness of your lungs and the fullness of them. In time your breathing will naturally skew towards fuller breaths and your total lung capacity will increase too. Of course, there are times where emptier breaths are appropriate and we'll address those specific drills later.

Principle #4 - Conscious vs. Subconscious

Breathing is one of the few processes in the body that is done both consciously and unconsciously. As such it is described as being the gateway into the subconscious mind in many mystic traditions.

(Contrary to what many people say, it is not the only activity that is both. I would argue that many pieces of vision, from the blinking of the eyes to where they move and focus on, is done both with and without conscious thought. Thus, visualization processes are also a similar sort of gateway. You'll see the combo of breathing and visualization in many of the intention focused breathing exercises.)

We've just discussed the ideas of making breathing both deeper, fuller, and through the nose. This is practiced consciously throughout many of the exercises in this book. One of the aims is to practice them enough that they become habit, so that the unconscious continues to breathe in this way.

But that is only one of our goals. Many of the drills covered in this book can be used as adjuncts to, or even by themselves as, meditative practices.

As the gateway into the subconscious mind, it is also the gateway into the autonomic nervous system, which by many was thought of to be beyond our control. However, through certain breathing practices, as well as visualization, we can control many of these autonomic functions including heart rate, bleeding, even the immune system function.

Most people have heard stories of yogi's and other people doing the seemingly impossible, like stopping their heart beat or piercing their skin and not bleeding. The breath is the starting point for these feats.

More recent research surrounding Wim Hof, known as the Ice Man, proved how breathing exercises could actually activate the innate immune system in such a way as to fight E. coli bacteria[4]. This was not just in him, but in students he taught in less than one week, showing that this ability is attainable by anyone willing to practice it. As a leading champion of breath work, we'll discuss more on Hof's specific techniques later on.

In addition to controlling functions thought to be beyond our control, on a simpler level the breath is a way to change our state. That is why you'll see we can use our breathing for meditation and to become stronger, to increase our endurance as well as our flexibility. Different breaths are used to aim the human body in different directions. The body can be thought of as the subconscious and thus this makes a lot of sense. We can then consciously choose to change the subconscious.

Principle #5 - Anatomical vs. Paradox

This principle refers to your breathing in regards to moving your body. First of all, note that breathing is a movement. Muscles are at work in this process with every inhale and exhale.

Anatomical breathing is what happens naturally when you move. Hence it is also called natural breathing. The idea is that your movements will either be opening up space or closing it down within the lungs. As such, air will naturally flow in or out. Other movements support the movement of inhaling and exhaling, and thus less effort is needed to breathe. This is an important concept especially in the application of endurance, as it is a relaxed way to breathe.

The opposite of anatomical breathing is paradoxical breathing. It's called paradoxical because you are going to breathe in contrast to how your body is actually moving. This becomes important mostly in strength related movements. The purpose of it is in creating pressure for added support and stabilization.

Think of doing a heavy barbell squat. If you breathed anatomically, as you did the squat you would breathe out as you descended, because your torso would constrict in space. Yet with hundreds of pounds on your shoulders this would not be a good idea. Instead, you could hold your breath, or actually breathe in as you descend in order to create the pressure in your abdominal wall and torso to support the weight. Then as you ascend, you might also hold the breath, or you could breathe out, possibly in a pressurized manner. This is paradoxical breathing and all of these methods will be covered later.

To contrast this, go ahead and do a couple of bodyweight squats right now. Without the weight, paradoxical breathing is not necessary. You can allow the squat, especially at rock bottom, to press air out of the lungs, and allow it to flow back in as you come back to standing fully erect. This is anatomical breathing.

Neither of these methods are wrong. They are just different applications. Even within the same exercise, there are times to do one and times to do the other. It depends on the desired outcome and what will best help you to get there.

Understanding the difference between these two and then being able to use them when you move is key. This is important for any movement from weightlifting to dance, martial arts to sports, and beyond. Technique surrounding these ideas will be fully explored later, but it is introduced here so you understand it early.

Principle #6 - Cadence and Speed

The last principle we'll be discussing here is that of cadence or speed in breathing. Obviously, there is no one correct way to breathe, but how fast or slow it is will depend on what you are doing. The four different parts of each breath.

1. Inhale
2. Space between inhale and exhale
3. Exhale
4. Space between exhale and inhale

In some of the following drills, like box breathing, each of these four phases will be spelled out directly. In that exercise each leg is done equally, hence the box, which seems balanced, but really places the emphasis on the spaces between inhaling and exhaling, which are typically not emphasized.

In others, sometimes the spaces between inhaling and exhaling doesn't really exist. In other drills sometimes one of the phases is emphasized over the others. This allows us to get more of the effects that that one piece brings.

According to Chinese medicine, the inhale is considered more of a yin activity, while the exhale is considered more yang.

As you breathe, within the bronchi the gases diffuse into the blood in a process called gas exchange, with CO_2 leaving the body and O_2 coming in. Getting more oxygen into your system, which lessens the ratio of CO_2, serves to raise the blood pH, making it more basic or alkaline. Of course, this all occurs within a fairly narrow range, but the results are measurable. Normal range is around 7.4 for the blood, but deep breathing can bring it up to around 7.75. Forget about an alkaline diet, just breathe differently! One of the benefits of this is that when you're in those more alkaline range the cells are better at producing ATP which means more energy.

(This is also why people breathe into paper bags when hyperventilating, a speedy inhale and exhale. In these cases, they have become too alkaline. The bag traps more of the exhaled CO_2 which is then breathed back in, helping to acidify the body. Beyond panic attacks, this method sometimes is used for with migraines, hiccups, nausea, asthma and more.)

The drills that do point out a specific cadence are great to get started with, and for the desired effects they may achieve. That being said, once you have practiced different speeds and cadences you'll realize that you can work with any of them you choose. I highly recommend playing around with these to find what may work best for you.

APPLICATIONS
of
Breathing Exercises

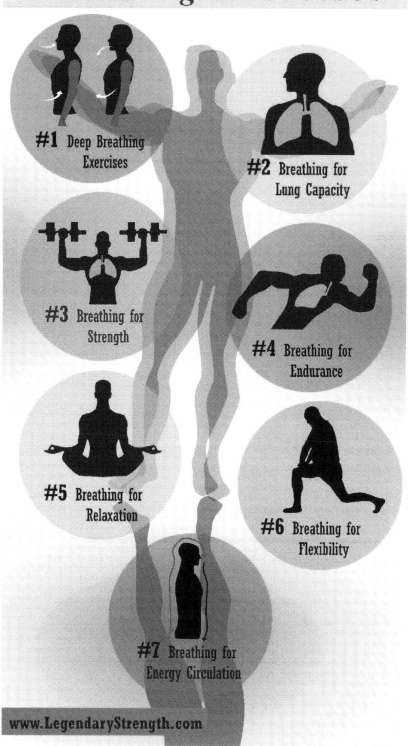

#1 Deep Breathing Exercises

#2 Breathing for Lung Capacity

#3 Breathing for Strength

#4 Breathing for Endurance

#5 Breathing for Relaxation

#6 Breathing for Flexibility

#7 Breathing for Energy Circulation

www.LegendaryStrength.com

Applications of Breathing

"By proper practice of pranayama all disease is eradicated.
Through improper practice all diseases can arise."
Swami Svātmārāma in the Hatha Yoga Pradipika

Now that we've covered the principles of breathing these can be put together in a number of different ways towards specific aims. Instead of just throwing a huge list of breathing exercises at you, this organization will help you to see how breathing can be used for a multitude of functions beyond just keeping you alive. For the purposes of this book I've divided breathing into seven different applications.

As categories these are all generalities. Some of the exercises could be used for multiple purposes. And some certainly could be put into multiple categories. But by breaking them up in this way you'll can get an idea of how they might best be used.

The seven categories, which you can see pictured on the previous page are:

1. Deep Breathing Exercises
2. Breathing for Lung Capacity
3. Breathing for Strength
4. Breathing for Endurance
5. Breathing for Relaxation
6. Breathing for Flexibility
7. Breathing for Energy Circulation

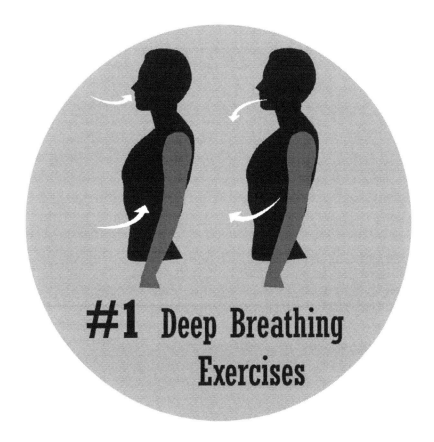

#1 Deep Breathing Exercises

"He lives most life whoever breathes most air." - Elizabeth Barrett Browning

Our first series of breathing exercises focuses on deeper and fuller breaths primarily. The purpose of these is to engage the lungs more than is normally done in regular breathing. This is the starting point, from which other forms of breathing for more specific reasons begins. If you've never focused on your breathing before, this is where you want to start.

Many of these when practiced consciously, will also begin to automatically help you to breathe deeper and more fully even when you're not consciously practicing. The habitual use of deep breathing is one of the goals we're after. It's great to breathe deeply each day in a routine, but if your breathing is shallow and empty the rest of the day, it can only help so much.

Mighty Atom Breathing Exercise

Joseph Greenstein, aka The Mighty Atom, who is one of my favorite old-time strongmen and a huge inspiration to me, was one of those people that didn't start out strong. In fact, he wasn't supposed to even survive as a child as he was so sickly. But he did, and at one point he ran away to join the circus. There he was mentored by the strongman and wrestler known as Volanko.

As described in the book, *The Spiritual Journey of Joseph L. Greenstein*, which is well worth reading, Volanko began Joseph on an exercise program, the first exercise of which was a deep breathing exercise.

The boy inhaled thinly, exhaled an asthmatic wheeze, then coughed.

"Tsk, tsk...terrible. You cheat yourself, little friend. The air is free. Look, like this." Volanko sucked in air through his nose while bringing his hands together over his head. Then he exhaled through his mouth and pumped his arms, working his lungs like a bellows. "Breathing is life, Yosselle. Without air, the fire dies. Now try again."

The boy tried to imitate him, and Volanko close one eye with a pained expression as his emaciated valet pulled away. "No, no, you'll faint if you do that. Slowly...relax..." The boy tried again. "Yes, more like that."

"How long do I have to do this?" the boy asked gasping.

"For the rest of your life," Volanko replied.

The story goes on to tell how Volanko instructed him in breathing. The following exercise can absolutely be done as described using the buckets, or other forms of weights. But even without those objects, simply raising your hands in the same manner, along with deep breathing, is a phenomenal exercise.

Little Joseph held a bucket in each hand, starting out by his legs. As he took a deep breath in, through the nose, the arms would rise out to the sides and come overhead. The reason buckets were used is that each day a handful of sand was added to each one. It was an imperceptible weight increase, but over time it began to add up. This is a great example of using micro progressions in training. Thus, along with the benefits of deep breathing here, there was muscular work on the arms and shoulders. The arms are lowered with an exhale through the mouth.

There isn't a mention of how many repetitions were done of this exercise each day, besides him struggling to do just ten reps in the beginning. I imagine it was typically somewhere in the range of twenty to fifty breaths and bucket raises like this.

The pace on this exercise is generally fairly slow. Inhale on the way up, pause for a moment, exhale on the way down, pause for a moment, and repeat. The key is that the arms are raising and

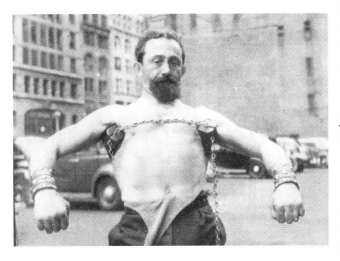

falling at the same pace as the breath. By the top of the movement you should have a full breath. By the bottom your lungs should be near empty.

You can use buckets if you'd like, but even just raising your empty hands overhead, this is a phenomenal breathing exercise to get started with.

Then if you want you can take your breathing much further, like breaking chains based on lung and chest expansion that the Mighty Atom regularly did, as pictured here!

Breathing with Arms Forward and Back

As was just covered, arms down to the sides up to overhead is a common method of deep breathing. But the arms can be similarly used in a variety of different positions as well. What follows is the favorite of strongman George F. Jowett, who, as it happens, was also a sickly boy, who grew up to become very strong.

You're going to start with your hands out in front of you, parallel to the ground. Inhale, opening the arms up until they extend to your sides and stretch them further back. Instead of just coming straight back, think of coming down behind a little which allows a little more of a stretch. You can even rise on the toes at the top of the movement, as Jowett preferred to do.

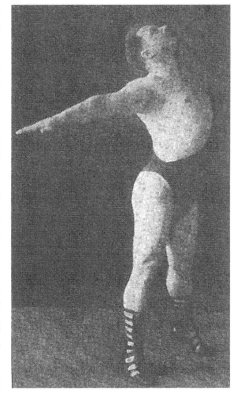

This is an anatomical breathing position. In the beginning, there is a slight constriction of the chest, which then is expanded as the arms move. You're especially stretching the shoulder blades, pinching them together, which opens up the lungs by giving you a big expansion of the chest. Bring the sternum forward, getting some thoracic spine movement in it as well.

Then exhale as you move the arms in front of your chest. You can actually cross your hands in front of your chest and this will help to squeeze the lungs more so. While doing so you can also flex your chest and make this sort of a dynamic resistance movement ala Charles Atlas. Repeat for ten reps or more.

Breathing with Forward and Back Bending

This breathing drill makes good use of anatomical breathing as well as improving the flexibility of your spine. You're only as young as your spine, thus it's a simple and great one to start your day with.

Stand with the feet about 18 inches apart. Exhale to start while standing straight. Now bend backwards bringing your arms back. You can bring them out to the sides or overhead. As you bend backward inhale fully. A brief hold with the breath and the body position can be done or you can reverse directions immediately.

Expel all your air as you bend forward at the waist, rounding the back fully. Reach for your toes or the ground. The legs should be keep loosely locked so that this bend also works the flexibility of the hamstrings. Again, you can pause with your breath and body position at the bottom or immediately reverse it.

A full inhale and exhale with a back and forward bend constitutes one rep. Repeat for ten reps or more. Pictured here is J.P. Mueller doing this exercise.

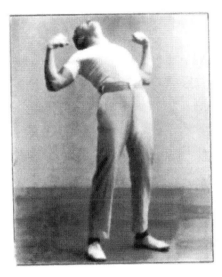 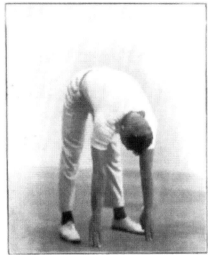

Full Tidal Breathing

Maxick was another strongman that grew up weak, but through proper breathing and exercise became strong. Are you detecting a pattern here? It seems that many of the weak ones placed even more emphasis on breathing than the naturally strong.

In some of the works by Maxick, he talks about the fallacies that people think of when they say deep or diaphragmatic breathing. What they do is they push out their stomach in order to breathe. But the simple distention of the stomach doesn't actually aid in breathing so much. What looks like stomach distention should naturally be a part of the diaphragm moving.

But there is much more to deep breathing than just the diaphragm too. Maxick, and his partner Monte Saldo, talk about this as "full tidal breathing". In addition to the diaphragm, the shoulder blades, intercostals and other muscles are used to expand the lungs. In practicing muscle control movements, this expansion can become much bigger, thus allowing even more room for the lungs to breathe.

The following is an excerpt from *Maxalding* by Monte Saldo:

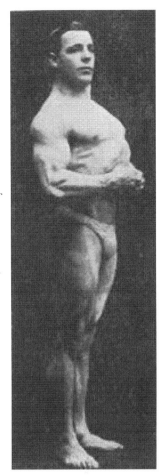

"Maxalding lung-capacity is not gained by forced deep breathing, but by the use of ingenious exercises such as [the following exercise], wherein by a simple manipulation, the shoulder blades are used as a pair of hands might be, to stretch and loosen the muscles surrounding the thorax. So effective in the thoracic movement - independently of the lungs - that Maxalding is used with great benefit by persons suffering from emphysema, because the action of the lungs can be replaced to a considerable extent by the voluntary expansion and contraction of the thorax. Air can thus be drawn into - and expelled from the lungs, in appreciable volume."

This breathing exercise should be done standing when starting out and can be done with the arms to the sides or the hands on the hips. Try both and see which one you prefer.

Begin to breathe in and think of spreading the lats, not by flexing the latissimus dorsi muscles, but by spreading the shoulder blades to the outside, in the opposite direction of what was done in the breathing with arms forward and back exercise. Spreading, not pinching. Think of breathing into the thoracic region, the middle of the spine, and even spreading or expanding the ribs apart.

Continue to breathe into this area of your back, as you spread the muscles, and now add in using your diaphragm more. Notice how much deeper of a breath this can become than just breathing low and forcing your stomach out. Recall that most of the mass of the lungs is in the back, and it makes sense that this allows more room to breathe.

Exhale as you reverse the shoulder blade movement and now pinch them together. Once you've done this a few times you can even stop consciously breathing and allow the anatomical movement to take over. It won't be as big of a breath as before, but you'll notice just how much air comes in from the space created in this movement. Repeat for ten reps or more.

After having practiced this exercise, you'll see why just using the diaphragm is not enough for full breathing, but the entire torso is in use. This is full tidal breathing. With more practice, and greater use of all these muscles, you'll expand your lung capacity.

Abdominal Vacuum

The abdominal vacuum is one of my favorite breathing exercises. It is quite a bit different than most as the way it is done involves not breathing in deeply but exhaling as fully as possible. It's suitable to cover this right after talking about Maxick and Monte Saldo because it is one of the best muscle control exercises there is.

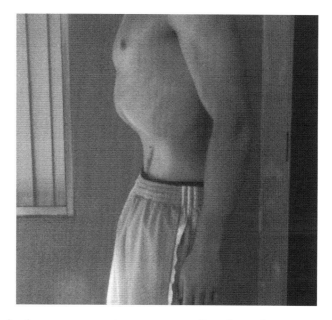

It is called the abdominal vacuum, or just vacuum for short, because you are blowing out as much air as possible to create a vacuum effect in your lungs. The diaphragm raises upwards, thus pulling your internal organs and the abdominal wall with it.

The effects of doing this are several fold. First of all, this exercise acts like wringing out the sponge that is your lungs, squeezing out a good amount of the residual air that normally stays inside. Thus, it allows for an exchange of that stagnant air for fresh air. Sometimes a smoker, when doing this, will see smoke come out on the first rep, as some residual smoke had just sat there stagnant!

This exercise also acts as a massaging movement to your internal organs and lymph. Your organs normally don't move that much, but through this movement, they get moved around a bit which may help with their function slightly. There's also a large amount of lymph tissue and fluid in the gut, as that is where most of our immune system is situated to deal with digestion. Unlike blood, the lymph system has no pump, and is only moved by movement. The vacuum works directly on this area, thus getting all that lymph moving. This is very important for immune system health.

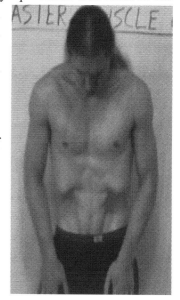

Speaking of moving the gut, most people tend to get old food stuck in the walls of the intestines. The vacuum also helps to get this stuff moving out as an aid to peristalsis. It's not uncommon for people to lose some of their spare tire by doing this exercise, not because it spot reduces the fat on your waist, but helps to clear up the waste on the inside. It can be said to help reduce your waist/waste.

Lastly, this exercise can be a fun one to do, with more advanced progressions that bring in more muscle control action. These include

"The Rope", as well as single sided abdominal isolation, where the abdominal rectus muscles, or just some of them, are flexed while in the vacuum position. But for now, we'll just stick with the main exercise. If you'd like to pursue those, check out the works of Maxick, other muscle control experts, or the *Master Muscle Control* video course I put together.

Now that we've talked about all the benefits it's time to learn how to do the vacuum. It is important to note that you may not see a pronounced vacuum effect the first time you try this exercise. Keep at it and over time you'll be able to achieve a greater vacuum. Having lower body fat certainly helps in achieving a more noticeable effect too. But even if you can't see it, as long as you do the exercise correctly, you'll be gaining the benefits.

It is not recommended to do this exercise within an hour of eating. Doing so can be uncomfortable. The best time to practice the vacuum is first thing in the morning. To aid in eliminations even more, do it after drinking a glass of warm water.

Breathe all your air out completely, as much as you possibly can. It helps to bend over at the waist and put your hands on your knees. This anatomical position helps to exhale completely and you can even round your back and shoulders to aid it further.

After exhaling as much as possible draw up on your diaphragm. As this is a muscle that most people aren't use to moving consciously here's a couple of tips so you can get a feel for that. As you are bent over think of moving your upper body away from your hips. Having exhaled this should naturally begin to create that vacuum effect.

A common mistake is to suck in your stomach but that's not really what is happening here. The vacuum pressure, created by relaxing the diaphragm, is moving your stomach in rather than you purposefully doing so.

By practicing some of the other deep breathing exercises you'll gain the feeling of your diaphragm, building that mind-muscle connection, and thus will be able to do this exercise better. As I previously mentioned, keep practicing it and you'll achieve greater and greater effects with it over time.

Only hold the vacuum for a few seconds. It's not necessary to go beyond ten seconds, and more typically I just do about six. After the hold, inhale fully between reps. If you need to, breathe deeply a few times before starting the next rep. In total, you should do three to ten reps of the vacuum exercise.

Box Breathing

Box breathing is a specific form of cadenced breath. It is called box breathing because each leg of the breath, inhale, hold, exhale, hold, is the same length. Thus, if you drew it out in the number of seconds for each one turning 90 degrees for each transition, it would look like a box.

Box breathing is great for relaxation too, but I've put it in the deep breathing section because if you expand the time in each leg it takes deeper breathing to do.

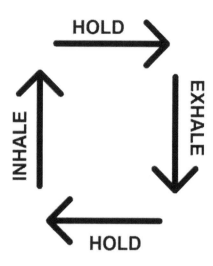

The starting point with box breathing is to do each leg for a four-count. Inhale for four seconds, hold for four seconds, exhale for four seconds, hold for four seconds, and repeat. Most people are not used to holding their breath after exhaling so that can be a little tricky at first, but becomes easier with practice.

You can do this with a fairly natural inhale and exhale or you can aim to fully inhale and fully exhale within those four seconds. The former keeps it more relaxing. While the latter makes it a stronger deep breathing exercise. By fully exhaling the hold afterwards becomes tougher too.

While this is a great drill to do just sitting or standing, I find that I like it best while moving. Start by walking. Instead of counting seconds, you can count steps. Thus, you start with a four step inhale, four step hold, and so on.

And you can take it still further running. Here, you might want to count every other step. This can become a good endurance challenge as the holds become increasingly difficult to do. A similar pattern, but without the holds, will be covered later as it will actually aid in your running.

In any of these different ways of doing box breathing, over time you can work to increase the length of each leg. Move to a six count, a ten count and beyond. The hold after the exhale will always be the limiting factor. If you're using this more for relaxation or meditation you'll want to keep it easily within your control. If you're aim is deep breathing though, keep working on extending that count.

Wim Hof Breathing Method

Wim Hof, the "Ice Man", has a fairly simple breathing technique that has many benefits. This is the foundation of how he, and the people he has taught, have done things like withstand cold exposure for long periods of time, as well as activate their innate immune system.

This breath is a focused fairly big inhale, but not completely full, then the exhale is just relaxed. I personally like to breathe in through the nose and out through the mouth on this, for the reasons previously covered, though Wim says either nose or mouth breathing works either way.

With the emphasis on the inhale you're getting more oxygen in your body, allowing the exhale to happen naturally. Keep repeating this for a recommended 30-40 breaths and you may notice yourself getting lightheaded or feeling different effects across your body. As will be mentioned later on, this is something that works great before doing various forms of breath holding.

While a simple breathing technique, as has been shown with recent scientific research, this can have profound effects. Wim's methods are worth exploring in more detail and you can find his full online course at http://legendarystrength.com/go/wimhof/

Breath of Fire

This method of breathing from yoga or pranayama is often done in a sequence, after other deep breathing exercises. Unlike most of them where breathing is slow, this one is quick. With the Breath of Fire you're basically using your lungs as a bellows, fueling the fire in the body.

This is deep breathing in that the diaphragm is pumping the action. But the cadence is very fast, typically up to two to three breaths per second, with an equal inhale and exhale both through the nose. As soon as you breathe in, you breathe out and repeat over and over again. When doing it you'll get into a rhythm and thus it can be made faster over time.

It is recommended to sit in a posture making sure that your spine is kept straight and tall. Your entire body is kept relaxed, the only movement coming from the belly and diaphragm.

The purpose of this breath is to energize the body. Literally think of fanning the flames. It quickly oxygenates the blood, helping to purify it. It also stimulates the nervous system and can help regulate glandular secretions. Quite a few other benefits are attributed to the breath of fire on top of these.

Recommended practice is to start with three minutes a day and then work up to going much longer, even fifteen to thirty minutes each day. Of course, this is one where people can get lightheaded and dizzy when starting out, so make sure to ease into it at a pace you can handle.

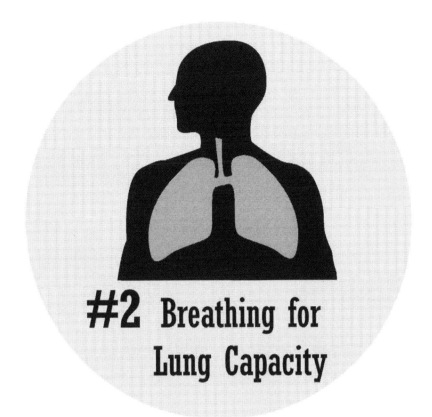

#2 Breathing for Lung Capacity

"To be good at breath holding it is crucial to be able to forget or dissolve time."
Stig Åvall Severinsen, 4-Time World Freediving Champion

Deep breathing exercises will certainly build up your lung capacity to some degree, but the following exercises focus specifically on that purpose. It comes down to expanding how much you can take in on an inhale, and then being able to hold your breath with that.

As we saw earlier, building lung capacity is an anti-aging practice. Thus, these exercises should be done by anyone interested in health.

Furthermore, this is helpful if any sort of endurance work is part of your training regimen. Simply having greater lung capacity makes those exercises easier to do as you can basically get by with less breath. I find that working on these is a great next step after practicing deep breathing exercises.

Segmented Breathing

Earlier in this guide, we talked about shallow versus deep breathing. In this exercise, we split the lungs up into three segments and breathe into, and out of each, in sequence. This ends up giving a similar effect as the full tidal breathing, but with a different approach.

I first experienced this in a yoga pranayama class, and found it to increase lung capacity better than just breathing fully into the lungs, as it helps to expand the different areas better by focusing in on them. Since that time, I have used it more for this purpose.

This can be done in a more relaxed manner, not filling the lungs as full as possible, but then the purpose changes more to that of relaxation and deep breathing. This is fine, just a different purpose than covered in the steps below.

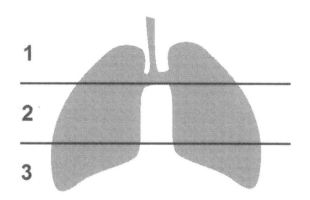

It helps to think of your lungs being split into a high, middle and low section. After some practice with this you can basically feel an imaginary line from one area to the next, thus filling in what feels like only that single section at a time. Of course, air is not just going into that one segment with each breath, but visualizing it helps the function of the drill.

Breathe into the high section of your lungs, expanding the upper chest and back as well as the shoulders. Pause for a second. Breathe into the middle section of your lungs, expanding the ribs and shoulder blades. Pause for a second. Breathe into the low section of your lungs, expanding the diaphragm and abdominals. Pause for a second.

Now begin the exhale in reverse order. Exhale the lower section of your lungs. Pause for a second. Exhale the middle section of your lungs. Pause for a second. Exhale the top portion of your lungs. Pause for a second. This constitutes one breath. Repeat for ten breaths or even longer as you like.

Don't worry if you're not getting the same amount of air volume with each segment. That is not the goal, so much as it is to bring awareness, and thus expansion, to the different areas of the lungs, as well as the surrounding musculature.

Also, feel free to experiment with the sequence of the segments. You could breathe into the top, middle, bottom, but then exhale in the same order, top, middle, bottom. Or you could start inhaling into the bottom, middle, top, then exhale reverse with top, middle, bottom.

Breath Holding

Did you know that breathing exercises can actually make you smarter? Anytime CO_2 increases within the blood supply, the body interprets that as a threat. Since the brain is one of the most critical parts of the body, it tends to send more oxygen up to the brain. Increased blood flow and oxygen helps with cognitive functions.

Of course, beyond that, another purpose of holding your breath is just to increase the lung capacity by itself.

The simple exercise to start breath holding is to just breathe in and hold it. Hold for as long as you are comfortable, and when it's a stress to go any longer, breathe out. This does come with a couple of warnings though. Obviously, if you went too long, you could black out and possibly injure yourself, so it is best to stop short of where your body enters panic mode. Further, if you have heart disease, high blood pressure or other conditions you would want to ease into doing this slowly, just like with other forms of exercise.

There are some people that state breath holding is harmful. To me this is as ridiculous as saying either the inhale or exhale is detrimental. If breath holding was harmful to your health, freedivers would all kick the bucket at young ages. But that is not the case.

One of the reasons I like breath holding is that it is progressive, and what gets tracked, gets improved. It's great to do deep breathing exercises, but sometimes seeing your progress in them is tough to do. Here, it is an easily trackable measure of time.

Beyond the first few times you try breath holding, and to take this further, it isn't enough to just breathe in and hold. Before the hold it is helpful to over saturate your body with oxygen, which then allows you to do the hold much longer. I have been playing with several different forms of this.

The first is to basically hyperventilate. Breathe in and out quickly and repetitively. This can make you light headed so don't overdo it. After you have done this for a little while, take a big inhale and then begin your hold. The other method is the Wim Hof method which was covered before in the deep breathing section.

In world record breath holds, they often do similar methods as these. Some of these involve breathing in pure oxygen. Recall that Tom Sietas went over 22 minutes in a breath hold, but first hyperventilated on pure oxygen. Unless you plan to go for that record yourself, I think just breathing in normal air is fine for our purposes. Normal breathing holds under water, without the use of pure oxygen, are closing in on the 12 minute mark. Why underwater? That is covered shortly.

Stig Åvall Severinsen, who formerly held the record several times, was measured by researchers in Denmark and was found to have a total lung capacity of over fourteen liters. This is more than twice as much as the average lung capacity of five to seven liters. This proves lung capacity can most definitely be increased.

The most important aspect of a long breath hold is the ability to relax both physically and mentally. In Severinsen's book *Breathology,* he details several methods that can help you to go longer. As you practice you will want to experiment to find what works best for you and this may involve some changes over time.

- Sitting or even lying down will allow you to relax the most.
- Breathing before the hold should involve exhaling through the mouth which opens the alveoli up to absorb more oxygen.
- Before doing your inhale, take a big yawn which helps to relax the body.
- After your big inhale, press down on your thighs, which shifts the diaphragm, lowering the pressure in your lungs, thus allowing you to be able to breathe in more.
- While holding your breath get in touch with your heartbeat and focus in on it.
- While holding think of pleasant memories or other things that serve to relax you. Do not focus on the clock.

I tend to try to keep my mind clear while I do these holds, but other people may find that the time passes more quickly if they distract themselves by thinking about something else.

Having some sort of timer is useful so you can actually make this progressive like any other physical training. Start with a minute, if you can. If you need to start with less than that, that is fine too. Then just add a few seconds here and there. Eventually you'll be doing it for several minutes. My personal record, at the time of writing this, is four minutes and fifteen seconds. However, it is important that you don't watch the clock, as it tends not to be relaxing to do so.

I have also noticed that there seems to be a warm up effect that is important. First of all, this is also great to do after other deep breathing and lung expanding exercises. They act to stretch and ready the lungs for this hold. When I started working on breath holds, as I increased the hold I did each morning by five seconds, I could just do one breath and that was it. But now, as I start to go longer, I find that two or three shorter holds before I go for a new record, seems to work better. You can think of it as a max effort lift, in a sense, and you wouldn't just jump into doing that without some preparation.

Exhale Holds

You can also hold your breath after an exhale instead of after an inhale. Of course, this is harder to do and you won't go as long. It is the method recommended by Wim Hof, after doing his breathing method covered earlier. In this case, it is not a full exhale, but a natural exhale, so there is still some air left in the lungs. Still this is tougher than holding after a big exhale. The point in this is that more oxygen should already be circulating in your blood from the previous breathing, allowing you still to hold for a while.

Feel free to experiment with a relaxed exhale and a full exhale and note the difference. The full exhale will definitely be harder, but working on it may help the other holds too.

This is a great way to switch up how you practice breath holds. For a while, I got stuck at holding my breath with a personal record of three minutes and forty-five seconds. After I hit this mark, I couldn't seem to surpass or even reach it again. But then I started practicing exhaled holds. As I built my time up in these to three minutes, I felt my abilities had grown. Then I switched over to a full inhale hold and immediately I exceeded the mark with four minutes and fifteen seconds.

The Diving Response

Breath holds can be made easier when we look at the benefits of what is known as the mammalian dive reflex. This reflex is very strong in aquatic mammals, but is also present in humans, just to a lesser degree.

Upon submersion in water, the heart rate slows down roughly ten to twenty-five percent. Vasoconstriction occurs as blood is shunted away from the periphery and into the organs, most notably the brain and heart.

But it doesn't take going fully underwater to activate this reflex. Just cold water on the face alone is sufficient as receptors on the face send signals to the brain which activate this autonomic response. The response also appears to be in relation with the temperature of the water. The colder the water, the more of an effect it has.

So, if you want to take your breath holds further, you have a few options. You can submerge yourself completely in a pool, dunk your face in a bucket of water, or allow cold shower water to hit your face. I would recommend you work on breath holds on dry land as well, and in this way, to compare the two.

Another option, though not quite as effective, is to soak a rag in cold water and then place it on your face while doing breath holds. In my experience this does seem to have some effect, while being easier logistically to do than other methods.

There is another dive response that is not as well-known and has only come to light in recent studies[5]. During breath holding, the spleen contracts, seemingly to squeeze its store of extra red blood cells into the circulatory supply, to provide oxygenation to tissues. This response is delayed in comparison to the dive reflex but seems to start occurring within thirty seconds.

It doesn't seem as if there is anything you can do to increase or utilize this effect beyond what will automatically occur. However, there's a good chance that this effect may be healthy for the spleen and in some way assist in its functioning.

Exercise with Breath Holds

Having just talked about the dive response and holding your breath, now as we talk about exercise, swimming is the natural choice. Of course, there are many varieties of this, some of which involve extended breath holding, while others involve breathing at certain intervals while swimming. I personally have not done a whole lot of swimming, so I'll leave that to people that do. I do believe it can be great exercise, and training for the breath too; I just haven't done a lot of it myself.

Instead, I want to focus on other exercises, along with breath holds, which I do have more experience with. The hard part of this is that when you are moving while holding your breath, you are expending energy thus you need more oxygen and you need to clear out that CO_2. It's much harder to hold your breath exercising rather than just sitting there not doing anything.

One common exercise I use for this purpose is the bodyweight squat. As before, you can start with pre-breathing for the breath hold, but now when you hold your breath you begin doing the exercise. I recommend squatting to rock bottom on each rep instead of parallel, assuming you have the flexibility to do so.

Whereas before you focused on time of the hold, here you focus on how many reps you can do instead. In my experience 20 reps in the bodyweight squat is a decent starting point. I've recently just hit 40 reps and am aiming for 50.

This can be done with a variety of different exercises like pushups, situps, pullups, kettlebell swings and many more. Most often it is with bodyweight exercises, but feel free to experiment with others if you choose. Wim Hof recommends the pushup for this purpose.

These exercises can be done with the full inhale, partial exhale, or even complete exhale.

Another option, and this one you need to be extra careful with, is holding inversions while holding your breath. My favorite is the headstand. The reverse flow of gravity further drives blood to your brain, but it also amplifies the possibility of blacking out, so once again use caution. If you've never done headstands before, I would do those without any sort of breath holding first to make sure you're safe and confident before trying to hold your breath in that position.

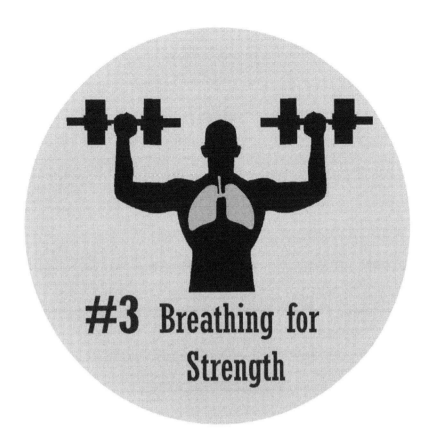

#3 Breathing for Strength

"All bodily power comes from the breath." – Strongman Volanko

Breathing is not just for relaxation or endurance. When we change up how it's done, it can very easily be used in order to become stronger. As with everything else, there is a time and a place for these techniques. What is covered here is really those movements that are more towards the max strength side of the scale.

Many people, that have no training in these methods previously, can see a ten to twenty percent increase in strength immediately. Thus, if you wish to be strong, you must master these drills.

But some people take them overboard and use them with every movement or exercise they do. In my opinion, it should be done less often than that. The point I'm trying to drive home is that there are no right and wrong ways to breathe, but appropriate applications for each.

Tension Hold

One method of breathing to gain strength is actually not to breathe. While holding your breath during an exercise is typically something trainers will tell you to stop doing, there is a reason we do it. It works!

Holding the breath is the natural reflex we seem to have when under pressure. The reason for this is that it pressurizes the torso, thus aiding in stability. Whether doing a squat, deadlift, press, or any number of other movements, this can be a big help.

Of course, it does have limitations. It's certainly useful when you are under a big load and need that added stability. But if you're doing something like holding a handstand, or repping out pull-ups, you will need to breathe, at least eventually.

There is one caution with this, and the following exercise. The tension hold and pressurized exhale will cause a temporary spike in your blood pressure. If you have high blood pressure, you should consult your doctor before doing these moves. You would be better off focusing on the deep breathing, relaxed breathing, and other drills in this course. Those may work over time to lower your blood pressure, then these drills could be added back in.

While holding your breath does work if you're going for strength, the following exercise often works even better.

Pressurized Exhale or "TSSSSSS"

Holding your breath creates pressure. But you can actually create more pressure by exhaling in the following way. By forcing a little air out at a time, your breathing muscles squeeze the air out. This also means they are tensing up even tighter than just with a hold.

The pressurized exhale is done through the mouth with the tongue on the roof of the mouth. The air will come out with a hissing sound. The goal is not to try to hiss, but instead to tighten the abdominal wall, so that the air is forced out with pressure. You create a virtual weightlifting belt that helps protect your body and also makes you stronger at the same time. Starting the sound off with a "T" rather than an "H" actually creates more pressure. Go ahead and try them yourself to feel the difference.

To protect yourself from the pressure going out the other end, you'll also want to squeeze the perineum or PC muscle. This is the same thing that is done in Kegels, drawing up on the pelvic floor, as if stopping yourself from taking a bowel movement. Here, it also protects you from hemorrhoids. This same 'locking' movement is done in many qi gong type exercises, so we'll revisit it later.

This can be done with any kind of moving exercise. It can also be done by itself. Matt Furey taught this as the Farmer Burns stomach flattener. Along with the vacuum and a few other abdominal movements it really can help to tighten up the stomach and develop your six pack by toning the muscles. As was addressed before, it's not about spot reduction of fat, but clearing out the intestines, and in this case adding tone to the muscles.

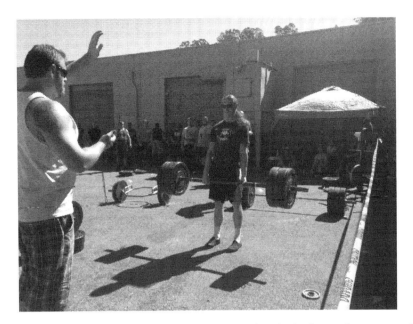

Pavel Tsatsouline is a big proponent of this pressurized exhale in various exercises as taught in *The Naked Warrior* and his other books. By creating additional pressure in the abdominals and surrounding muscles, through an effect he calls irradiation, the added tension spreads to other muscles, including whichever ones you are working with. For instance, let's say you're doing a military press. If you exhale in this manner you're more stable, and the added pressure allows you to tense up your shoulders and arms more, thus exerting more strength.

This is a useful technique for strength. So, should you use it every time? In my opinion no. It is useful for grinding lifts. But another way to be strong is to explode. And you can't explode when you're tense. (But with the right timing you can do a pressurized exhale at the most appropriate moment.) Still for maximum explosion you must start from relaxation.

Further, it seems that people that practice this all the time tend to get tenser overall in their body and movements. Generally, for movement quality, that is not something we want. Therefore, yes you should learn how to use this and use it from time to time, when it is needed, but not exclusively.

Breathing Behind the Shield

In cases of exercise where you're constantly under load, longer than you can hold your breath, you will want to do what is often called breathing behind the shield. In this case, the "shield" is the tensed up abdominal wall. It is kept tense in order to keep your body stable for whatever exercise you are doing, whether that be a plank, handstand, hollow body position, yoke walk, farmer's walk, loaded carry, weighted supports or any number of other exercises.

In order to do this, you will be taking a more shallow and empty breath. You can't take as deep or full of a breath as you might normally do because it would disrupt your ability to keep tight. This can be practiced without actually doing an exercise. Simply tighten up your core musculature and breathe without too much movement occurring in your torso.

Doing this in the most efficient way will take practice. It will also depend on the exercise itself, the position you are in, the load used and how used to the exercise you are. Yet with practice over time you will still be able to breathe fairly deeply behind the shield. This aids in endurance in any exercise where you need to do so for longer durations.

To take this one step further you can actually weigh down your chest by doing something like a stone carry at chest level, or a rack walk with two kettlebells. These implements make it harder to breathe, thus developing the ability to breathe behind the shield even better.

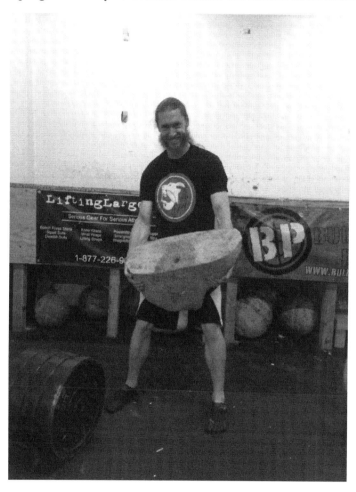

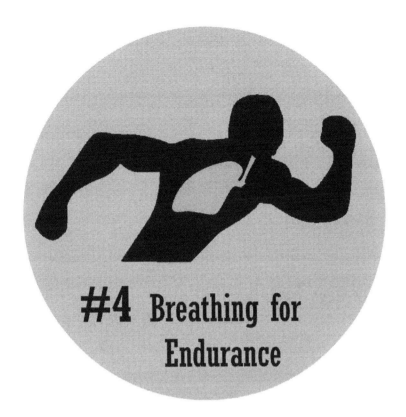

#4 Breathing for Endurance

"Good lungs are essential for anyone who is desirous of accomplishing anything in the endurance." – Earle Liederman

How you breathe when you are doing an endurance or conditioning exercise will make a huge difference in just how far you can go with it. It's important to note that with any exercise of this manner there can be two different aspects of endurance that will affect your performance.

One is your breath. And the other is your energy systems. Of course, these two are intimately tied to each other. The production of ATP in your cells works far more efficiently in the presence of oxygen. By practicing these breathing exercises you'll get better at both. Ultimately, though you may find the breath is not the hard part of any exercise you do, it becomes more limited by muscular fatigue.

That being said, these exercises are not focused on lung capacity. Those certainly help here too as they allow you to take more in and operate longer off of it. Instead, this section focuses in on the way you breathe in order to stay as relaxed as possible, thus expending less energy and oxygen. This is the key to great endurance. More tension means you'll tire out faster. Depending on what you're doing though you'll probably need some tension. Also, here you'll learn methods to catch your breath faster when you do run out of it.

A lot of this has to do with the rhythm of your breathing, working with anatomical breathing, as well as manipulation of the timing of each breath.

Breathing Rhythm for Endurance

Rhythm is a very important part of endurance. We already covered the difference between paradoxical and anatomical breathing. Regardless of which one you are doing, you want to have a rhythmic cycle. This is because when breath gets outside of control other things start to as well.

Typically for an exercise, you may have one in breath and one out breath per repetition. This is going to work well for most exercises. This is the simplest rhythm.

And the more you can really get into the rhythm of this breath with each rep the better you'll do. This is because you'll have to spend less time working on the breathing and can get into a better flow with the movement. Better flow typically means more relaxed, which once again, is critical for endurance.

For the most flow and relaxation, you will want the exercise to breathe you in its rhythm, but that will be covered more in the next point. If you're working with something hard or heavy, it may not be the best option though. The fact is, you can have rhythm with pressurized exhales too and even in breathing behind the shield.

With some exercises it won't be one cycle of breath per rep though. One exercise I like to point this out with is the kettlebell snatch. Depending on how you do this, it can be done different ways. The hardstyle snatch, which is more explosive, will have you breathe in before the bottom portion of the lift, creating abdominal pressure to protect the back, and then explosively out, a pressurized exhale, as you're exploding the bell to the top.

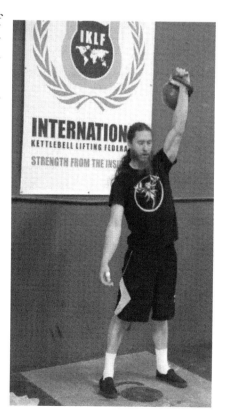

Contrast this to the girevoy sport, aka kettlebell sport, style of snatch. Here the goal is to last longer, as you're typically doing sets of ten minutes in length. You can't be maximally explosive, as that would tire you out. Here the breathing becomes anatomic. At the bottom you breathe out as your torso is bent and rounded. Then as you come up, using as much momentum from the bell as possible, and elastic recoil from your body, your chest opens and you breathe in.

While these are different, and for different purposes, they still have pretty much the same rhythm. One breath in and one breath out per rep, it's just inverted in timing, and from tension to relaxation.

A few years back I set out on the goal of snatching a 24kg or 53 lb. kettlebell 300 times in ten minutes. This is pretty close to full speed for the entire time frame and a very tough challenge. What I found was that I could not just breathe once per rep. It didn't allow for enough oxygen to keep that pace for that length of time as there were small periods of breath holding involved. What I needed was to be breathing in and out the whole time.

That is when I came up with what I call two-cycle breathing. All that means is doing two breaths per rep. There is both an inhale and exhale on the way up, and an inhale and exhale on the way down. This was the breathing style that ultimately allowed me to hit that goal. And snatches aren't the only thing you could do it in.

Let's talk about running. You will want to develop a rhythm with your breathing in line with your steps. Once again this will allow you to flow better with the movement. To inhale on one step and then exhale on the next will be too short of a breath. Instead, you will breathe in for a number of steps. I recommend starting with four. Then you exhale for the same number. Thus inhale for four steps, exhale for four steps and repeat. There is no breath holding in this, as there was with the box breathing mentioned earlier. Here, as soon as you finish one way, you reverse it.

Cycling, jumping rope, swimming, or anything else can be done in much the same way. Experiment and find what rhythm works well for you. Maybe it's every five steps or every six steps. You might even try making it an uneven rhythm, like four steps on inhale and five steps of exhale. Furthermore, counting the steps or the pace of your breathing can take your mind off of the exercise, and may enhance the meditative qualities of endurance exercises such as this.

The following picture of rowing movements, with different types of breathing, is taken from *My Breathing System* by J.P. Mueller. In the top figure, we see a rhythm that is anatomical and one breath per row. In the following pictures, we see two different types of two cycle breathing. Here you'll notice that different legs of the cycle are longer or shorter than the others, but there is still a certain rhythm involved with the breathing and movement.

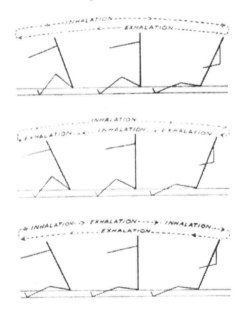

The main takeaway here is that there ought to be some sort of rhythm of breathing that coincides with the movement. Depending on the movement at hand, and your goal for it, this will have to change. A sprint is different than a jog, though they are both running, thus the breathing changes.

But by finding the appropriate breathing and syncing it up to the movement, you will have better endurance.

Be Breathed

This is a concept that I learned from Scott Sonnon. Be breathed implies that the movements themselves breathe you, rather than you breathing with the movement. It takes the preceding idea of rhythm and further expands upon it. You'll be using the anatomic breathing to actually cause air to go into and out of your lungs, without even trying to breathe. It may take a little getting used to at first but once you can do it, you'll be able to keep going and going.

Of course, this can only be done with certain exercises. You must rely on the contraction and expansion of the torso so that the movement breathes you. If you don't have that, this technique cannot be done in the same way. To get a feel for this, you can do a simple experiment that will show how this occurs.

Allow your breathing to relax so that you're not holding it, nor trying to inhale or exhale. Bring your chest up and your shoulders back. If you have let any pressure off your lungs and the surrounding muscles, when you do this, air should naturally flow in. The reason for this is because of the difference in pressure in the atmosphere's air and the air inside your body. By opening up the space by expanding the chest and shoulders there is more room for air in the lungs, thus a lower pressure, and so the air enters.

To contrast this, once again relaxing your breathing muscles so you're not causing it to happen, round your back fully and bring the shoulders forward. By closing the space, air should naturally flow out. Now, go back and forth between these two positions: chest up and shoulders back, to back rounded, shoulders forward. As you do it, the movement will cause breathing to occur for you.

That is a simple way to first experience being breathed. Still there's not a whole lot of movement in the torso, so these will be fairly empty breaths. The best way to get the full experience of being breathed is with the following rolling exercise.

Sit on the ground with your legs straight in front of you. Reach forward as if touching your toes and round your back. Notice that your lungs naturally exhale. Then reverse the movement and air starts to come in. Keep going backwards, rolling onto your back, allowing your legs to come up and reach behind you. At this point, your air will have been exhaled. This is like the plow movement in yoga except you're not going to hold it. Once the feet hit the ground, or as far as they go as your flexibility allows, roll back. As you come back to sitting, you will be inhaled. This is one repetition and it's important to note that there is a two-cycle breath per rep here.

To recap: bend forward allowing the exhale, come back to sitting allowing the inhale, roll onto back, exhale, and roll back to sitting, inhale. At both ends of the movement, forward and back, your torso is constricted, and it opens up in the middle portion.

In the beginning, take the movement fairly slowly. It is important to keep the lungs relaxed so that they can breathe for you. As you repeat more and more reps, note that you can increase or decrease the speed and the breathing will follow.

Because of the rhythm and the relaxation, after a couple of minutes, you can really get into the flow of this movement. For those reasons, it's great for the flexibility in the toe touch and plow position too.

You should be able to do this movement for a long time and never get out of breath with it. If you are getting out of breath then you're are tensing up and not properly allowing the movement to breathe you.

Other movements don't tend to breathe you as much as this one does, but after practicing this, you can see where it occurs in some movements. With a bodyweight squat or a kettlebell swing, the movement can breathe you. Chances are, unless you add more rounding of the back and extending of it than is typical, you will not get a full breath with each rep though. Still, this gets you use to letting the movements at least aid in natural breathing and thus can allow for better endurance.

Catching Breath Faster

This next exhalation tip, I got from Jon Haas, in his own breathing course, *Evolve Your Breathing*. This isn't so much how you breathe in an exercise, but what you do after you've done an exercise to help catch your breath better. It is focused on the exhale.

If you're breathing hard after an exercise, instead of just huffing and puffing, what you want to do is extend the exhale just a little bit longer than the inhale. By doing so you can clear out CO_2 faster, lowers your heart rate and blood pressure, all of which helps to catch your breath more so.

The reason that this can help is not really that you need more oxygen, but because there is too much CO_2 in your lungs. Furthermore, by extending the exhalation, you're actually going to relax the body a bit more.

As you do this, allow the inhale to happen naturally, from the recoil after exhaling deeply. You may even apply this to some forms of endurance, extending that exhale a little bit longer while you're actually doing the exercise, assuming it fits into the rhythm.

Lung Reenergizer

The lung reenergizer is an odd breathing technique that I picked up in my studies of energy medicine. It is based off of flushing the lung meridian. I note a distinct difference when I use it and when I don't in catching my breath. Others who I have taught it to have noticed the same thing.

The lung meridian is an energy channel that runs from the top outside, or superior lateral side, of the pectoral muscle, slightly up the shoulder than down the arm off the thumb. See the picture for details.

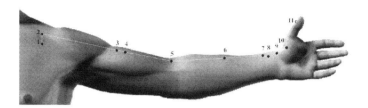

In flushing a meridian, you go backwards on it one time, than forward three times. The pathway of the meridian is traced physically with the opposite side hand. Think of the middle of your palm as moving the energy in the meridian. Here you'll do one arm and then the other. Doing so is kind of like working on the plumbing of your energetic system.

I do this with a certain method of breathing and I always note that I have caught my breath a bit more by the end of it. Breathe in as you start at the thumb and run up the meridian backwards. Then reverse directions and exhale as you move down the arm. Inhale again, starting at the pec and trace down the meridian while exhaling. Repeat that last step once more. So you trace backwards on the meridian once and then trace down it in the proper direction three times.

After you finish with one arm, do the other. Do this after any set of an endurance exercise. For further benefits make the exhale just a little bit longer than the inhale as covered in the previous point. Note your breathing before you do the lung reenergizer and then after it and you should note a strong difference. Although you may have caught your breath significantly you'll probably still notice your heart beating ferociously.

Breathing Ladders

A ladder, when it comes to exercise, is doing progressively more reps in each set. For instance, let's say you're doing pullups. You start with one rep then take a short break. On your next set, you do two reps then rest. Then three reps and rest. And so on. So, it can look like this 1,2,3,4,5,6,7,8… as far as you can go. This can also be done with other formats besides just adding a single rep at a time. You could do it by doubles or fives so 2,4,6,8,10 or 5,10,15,20 for instance.

Breathing ladders, which I first heard from Dr. James Heathers, are a modification of this idea where the breath is used as the main point of focus. You do the exercise breathing as you would normally while doing it, but your rest period is only as many breaths taken to match the number of reps you just did. So, one rep, one breath, two reps, two breaths, three reps, three breaths and so on.

You can do this with all sorts of different types of exercises. Squats, kettlebell swings, pull-ups, push-ups, hanging leg raises, deadlifts and many more will all work.

Doing this forces you to focus on deep breathing and controlling your breath to work your endurance and breathing capacity in a bit of a different manner than normal. Ultimately, you will likely be stopped not by muscular fatigue, but by running out of breath. I recommend trying to do it all breathing through the nose, at least as far as you can, before switching to mouth breathing.

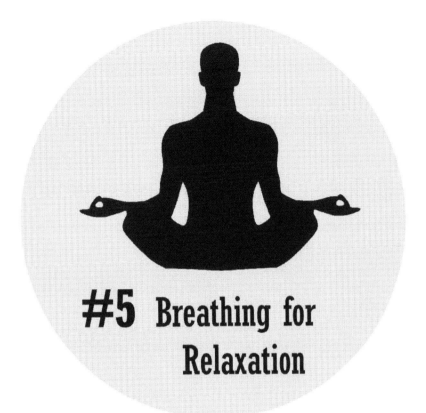

#5 Breathing for Relaxation

"Feelings come and go like clouds in a windy sky. Conscious breathing is my anchor."
- Thich Nhat Hanh

The breath is not only key for strength and endurance, but also for relaxation too. In fact, the main way in which it helps with endurance is by helping to keep the body as relaxed as possible.

The following exercises could also be taught as deep breathing exercises, but instead I'm showcasing them as relaxation breathing exercises. Remember, these are not hard and fast categories, but instead just different ways of categorizing that can aid us in thinking, and thus using breath work in different ways. Many of the exercises already covered can be used for these purposes too.

These exercises can be useful for different types of meditation. Starting any meditation practice with some deep breathing can be a useful way to relax and center your mind. That's not to say these are the only ways to do it, but simply breathing like this for an extended period of time can be a meditation in its own right.

Centering Breath or 6-2-7

This is commonly known as the centering breath, a specific cadence that is used in breathing, holding and exhaling. Of course, it's not the only method of centering yourself with breath so a more descriptive name of the 6-2-7 breath is also used.

This refers to inhaling at a six count, holding for a two count and exhaling for a seven count. With this breath, there is no hold after the exhale; you just go right back into inhaling. You could reverse it immediately though you may find a brief pause of less than a second more natural.

Without much holding, and with a slightly longer exhale than an inhale, this breath is great for relaxing and getting centered. It is slower than the average breath too. Repeat it for ten or more breaths and you'll find out for yourself. Repeat it for ten minutes or so, and you'll have entered an altered state for sure.

Alternate Nostril Breathing

Experts in yoga tell us that alternate nostril breathing helps synchronize both hemispheres of the brain. This is especially useful for those of us who get stuck in the logical, rational left-side thinking often. The left brain, right brain thing is really an oversimplification of how the brain works, but there is certainly some merit to it. Lots of other benefits are attributed to the method as well.

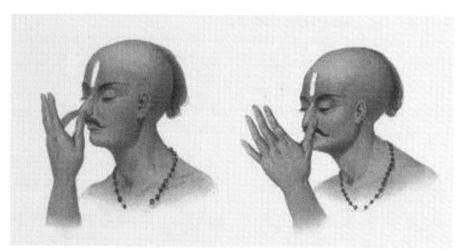

As the name indicates, you will be breathing in through alternating nostrils one at a time. As such, this involves breathing in and out through the nose.

While you could do this in any number of ways, there is a traditional hand position that I was taught. I use my right hand, but if you're left handed, you could simply mirror the position. Start with you palm in front of and facing your face. Your thumb will close your right nostril. Place the index and middle fingers on the third eye.

With the thumb holding the right nostril closed, breathe out with the left nostril. It is recommended to breathe out of the left nostril as the start to any alternate nostril breathing. Now inhale through the left nostril.

Place your ring finger over the left nostril, closing it. Remove the thumb from the right nostril. Exhale and then inhale through the right nostril. At this point, you've completed one full cycle which contains two full breaths. Move the thumb back over the right nostril and release the ring finger on the left and repeat. This is the hand position I use, but anyway you do it should provide the same benefits.

Repeat for as many breaths as you choose. I personally just do a few breaths, ten or so cycles, before my morning meditation practice. While I could go much longer, I can feel the calm centeredness from this exercise after just a few breaths. And since this practice is after other breathing exercises I do, I don't feel the need to keep going much longer. But that's just me. You may wish to do this for an extended period of time, as is often recommended.

Alternate nostril breathing can be combined with box breathing, the 6-2-7 count, or any other cadence of breathing you choose. Experiment and find what works well for you. The following progressive method, where a week or even a month was spent at each cadence, was outlined by Severinsen in his book.

Week	Inhale	Hold	Exhale	Hold	Ratio
Week 1	4 seconds	0 seconds	8 seconds	0 seconds	1:0:2:0
Week 2	4 seconds	4 seconds	8 seconds	0 seconds	1:4:2:0
Week 3	4 seconds	4 seconds	8 seconds	4 seconds	1:1:2:1
Week 4	4 seconds	8 seconds	8 seconds	4 seconds	1:2:2:1
Week 5	4 seconds	8 seconds	8 seconds	8 seconds	1:2:2:2

It Breathes Me from Autogenics

Autogenics is a method of getting the body to respond to verbal commands. Created by the German psychiatrist Johannes Shultz, this involves a daily practice of relaxing and repeating commands, not necessarily out loud, but thinking them, several times a day. The results were that people could learn to balance sympathetic and parasympathetic activity, ultimately helping with things such as blood pressure, immune function and more.

There are several different steps, including feeling the warmth and heaviness of the limbs. A few steps later, the breathing is focused on and that is what our attention is turned to here. I bring it up because it shows a different way of thinking about breathing.

Often when we are doing deep or relaxing breathing exercises we focus our conscious attention on breathing. This is useful in that we can change how we breathe from default. But in doing so we tend to also put effort into the breathing, in order to make it different.

In autogenics, the phrase "it breathes me" is used. Go ahead and breathe, while repeating this phrase with each in-breath and out-breath. Notice how thinking of the air itself breathing you, rather than you breathing it, changes the quality of your breath. Don't try to breathe slow, deep or fully but instead allow the air to breathe you. It's almost like the be breathed exercise except you're not relying on your anatomical position to breath you.

Try doing this for at least three minutes, and note your experience and how it is different from other exercises. Once again, this idea could be combined with a number of other breathing exercises.

Sharpshooter's Trick

The former exercises in this section are all about breathing to achieve relaxation. This final exercise is an application of the same. It is called the sharpshooter's trick, or the marksman's trick, as it is used in shooting, among other things.

The idea with this is that after you have exhaled, that's when the body is most steady, calm, and you're able to exert the most technical ability in many physical skills. You breathe out and in that pause before the next inhale begins, maybe one to three seconds, is the correct timing.

This is something you can experiment with anytime you are practicing a physical skill. If you're playing the piano or another instrument it won't be very helpful. But in similar things to taking a shot, where you need everything focused just for that moment, it can be very useful. For instance, I like to exhale and then hold my breath as I kick up into a handstand. As soon as I hit my position, I take the inhale and begin breathing behind the shield.

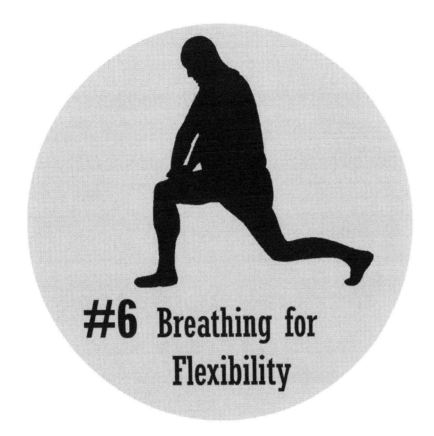

#6 Breathing for Flexibility

"Above all, learn how to breathe correctly." – Joseph Pilates

Beyond knowing the technical details of how to do a stretch, the breath is the most important part that will allow you to gain in flexibility. Through these two techniques you'll be able to go further, often instantly.

Besides applying them to a stretch, these breathing methods are no different from what you have already learned when breathing for strength and breathing for relaxation. Both becoming stronger as well as allowing the muscles to relax are important components needed for flexibility and thus we use breathing that functions for both.

Isometric Stretching

This technique goes by many names, sometime with specific variations, including PNF or proprioceptive neuromuscular facilitation, isometric stretching, or the hold and release method.

The breathing technique is really just a combination of things that you've already learned. Enter any stretch going near your maximum range of motion. While staying here inhale and hold while tightening up your muscles. The muscle or muscles that you're stretching should be flexed and you can also flex everything that is surrounding it. This can be an isometric push against the floor or whatever is involved in the stretch. While you do this, make sure that you stay at the same spot and don't go backwards in your stretch, as sometimes the body wants to do.

After holding for a few seconds, exhale, releasing all tension at the same time and sinking a little deeper into the stretch. Repeat this process a few times.

The great thing about this method is that by tensing the muscles isometrically you're actually building strength in this end range of motion. Flexibility is often limited, because you're not strong enough in that range. Your body won't let you go there for fear that you won't be able to get out.

The isometric squeeze is usually done for a short amount of time like three to ten seconds. An alternative, that requires you to breathe rather than holding the breath, is to go much longer.

In some cases, this is thirty seconds, or even up to a couple of minutes. The purpose of this is to tire the muscles out which allows you to go further. With tired muscles, they won't be as able to resist you going deeper into the stretch. While doing this, since you'll be tensing up the body, you're basically breathing behind the shield. Shallow breathing while you squeeze, but then the exhale, relaxing and releasing the exact same.

Doing this practice regularly helped me to achieve the full front splits.

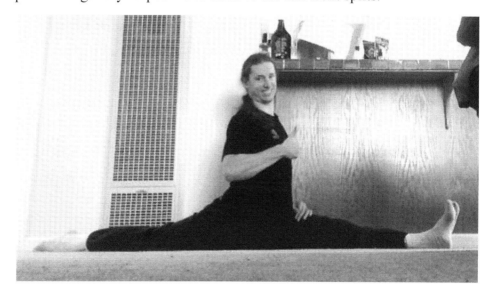

Breathing into Muscles

The previous exercise is like going in the opposite direction, tension, to force the direction you want, relaxation. In contrast, this technique goes straight after the relaxation. It does not involve purposefully tensing up like the previous one, but instead focuses your breath with intention and relaxation into the muscles being stretched. A stretched muscle is tense, even if you're not adding to it with an isometric push, and it is this tension that limits your ability to go further.

With a stretch, you feel a sensation that we call a stretch. Depending on what the flexibility exercise that you're doing and your depth into it, this stretch can become quite uncomfortable. It shouldn't be painful in the sense of causing damage, but certainly many people would describe it as such. Understanding the difference between sensation, discomfort, and pain is important in listening to your body.

For this method, while in any stretch you think of inhaling into the muscle being stretched as if directing the energy there. Then you exhale, and as before, and allow the muscles to relax. Here, you may sink further into the stretch, or you can repeat the slow inhale and exhale a couple of times simply focusing on relaxing the muscle further before going deeper.

This drill focuses on the mind-muscle connection, using the gateway of the breath. It is helpful to also visualize the muscles stretching and relaxing as well. Sometimes a metaphoric visualization like that of ice melting, the breath bringing in heat to do so, can aid even more so.

For any flexibility you're working on, a mix and match of these two techniques, even back to back, can be quite helpful. Of course, there are other flexibility methods like dynamic stretching that are worth incorporating as well.

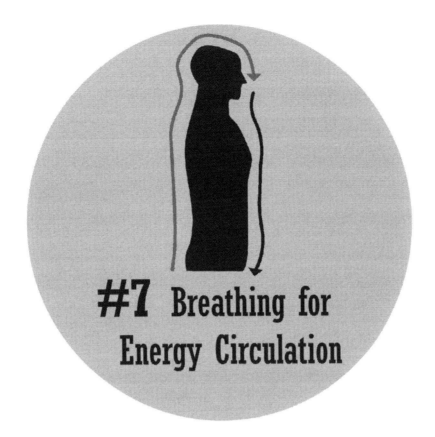

#7 Breathing for Energy Circulation

"Inhale, and God approaches you. Hold the inhalation, and God remains with you. Exhale, and you approach God. Hold the exhalation, and surrender to God." - Krishnamacharya

Now we start to get into the "woo-woo" area of breathwork. I say that tongue in cheek for a couple of reasons. Whenever we talk about energy or intention, many people turn off to the idea thinking it's not scientifically based. I believe that it is; it's just that science hasn't always caught up with it, although that is available if you look in the right places. Still, some people take these concepts a bit too far.

That all being said, because breath does allow us to tap into the conscious and subconscious, it also makes sense that it is a huge part of the border between the physical, and the more etheric; whether we talk about energy fields, or simply the mental and emotional aspects of human beings.

Also, I decided to call this category, breathing for energy circulation, as many of the drills involve the movement of energy. Truthfully, that's only part of it though. It could be called breathing with intention. Or instead of deep breathing, breathing to go deeper.

What is covered below are just a few starting points. This area could be explored in much further detail, and ultimately, I believe it's where the higher level of breath work will lead you. That being said, a lot can be done with just a few basic ideas so let's get started.

Intention and Direction of Breath

When doing any of the other breaths, your intention is typically involved. But in this exercise, we take it a step further, moving the intention beyond just breathing into the lungs. Although the lungs may be the extent of where the air gets to, except of course with the oxygen getting into the blood and then the blood circulating across the entire body, we can think of breathing into different areas. Perhaps, by doing breathing with intention like this, then the blood is "instructed" to oxygenate the area more.

This idea was done with the last flexibility exercise, but it has other applications as well. One purpose is to breathe even deeper than your diaphragm. Think of breathing into your feet and notice how this may change how grounded you feel. You can go even deeper than this. Breathe into the earth below you as if you are a conduit from which the earth can breathe through you.

If you have an injury in a certain area of the body, intention can be used. In an acute injury, you can martial the immune system and other repairing functions to the area. But this may be especially useful in the case of chronic injuries, where lack of circulation can be a piece of why it stays a chronic issue. Let's say you have a knee injury. Imagine you have a lung in the knee and breathe in and out of that.

This is likely to have great applications with several diseases too. Dr. Otto Warburg, who won the Nobel prize in 1931, stated, *"Cancer, above all other diseases, has countless secondary causes. But, even for cancer, there is only one prime cause. Summarized in a few words, the prime cause of cancer is the replacement of the respiration of oxygen in normal body cells by a fermentation of sugar. All normal body cells meet their energy needs by respiration of oxygen, whereas cancer cells meet their energy needs in great part by fermentation."*

This has led to various forms of alternative treatment with ozone therapy and the like. But what if we simply breathe into that area? Multiple studies have shown the effectiveness of visualizing white blood cells being more effective and thus achieving a greater immune system response[6]. I imagine that breathing into an area with a similar type of visualization would do just the same. It could mobilize circulation, immune response, energy and who knows what else to target whatever you're trying to target. I wouldn't advise someone to only do this in cases of cancer or other disease, but I think it could certainly be a helpful adjunct to several other treatments they're doing whether conventional or alternative.

In fact, we see that the immune system did respond better to E. coli bacteria in research done on Wim Hof and his students from doing breathing exercises. [4] It did not take years of training, only a few hours before his students achieved this effect.

An alternative format is to breathe in and out with the lungs but then send the energy and breath to the area of focus. You can accumulate the energy through breathing and then direct in in a sequence of steps.

You can breathe into a specific organ like the liver or the heart. By doing so you'll achieve a greater awareness of that organ. In ancient systems, the organs always stored emotions so these could come up through breathing processes like this as well. I like to think of each organ being its own intelligence and thus this is a great way to "communicate" with them. These days, there is a lot of talk about the gut and the heart as the other "brains" in the body, but what if that is true of each and every organ?

You can breathe into energetic pathways, like the meridians or into specific chakras, in much the same way. By keeping your focus in one area, this can't help but do be a meditative type of breathing.

You may have heard the saying that energy flows where intention goes. Here your intention is to go deeper. Remember in the beginning, where we talked about if you haven't used certain muscles before, like those surrounding the diaphragm, just by doing so, you're going to expand your awareness of that area and be able to use it better. Here, it is much the same, and thus can unlock more feelings and awareness around your energy, mental and emotional body.

An entire breath practice could be born out of these ideas. What would it be like to start your day by breathing into each organ, each meridian and each chakra each day? We covered a multitude of different possibilities just in this section. Take some time to explore these ideas for yourself.

Feldenkrais Breath

Moshe Feldenkrais was a genius in the area of somatic awareness. I have only begun to explore his work. In his book, *Awareness through Movement*, Feldenkrais details a few breathing exercises. Here is one of them:

> *"Now imagine the passage of the air as it enters your nostrils and goes to the back of your palate and into your windpipe. Think only about this point every time you breathe in, until all these parts are known and familiar to you. When this first section has become clear, follow the air in its passage from there to the right upper bronchi. Now go back to the nostrils; when these are familiar move on to the palate, all down the windpipe, to the space around the windpipe, to the air that flattens the lung against the walls of the chest, and is itself forced upward, down toward the floor, toward the shoulder and the armpit."*

Here, your awareness extends into much more minute detail on the air as you breathe it, and the different areas of your body that are touched by it. In doing so, you'll gain greater awareness on the movement of your breath. He goes on further to describe drills where you notice if you can feel the breath from the left nostril into the left lung. Then do the same with the right side. Both lungs are obviously going to fill up with air, but it's going to have a little bit of a different feel to it by doing it this way.

Work to blend the visual imagery with the feeling of the breath on both the inhale and the exhale. Perhaps even the breath can move around in your body while you're holding your breath. As synthesia is often a useful aspect of genius, in this case blending the visual and kinesthetic, being able to do this may be able to unlock deeper levels of ability.

Microcosmic Orbit

The microcosmic orbit is a breath and intention drill that is found in various qi gong and meditation practices. Its purpose is internally circulating the energy in the body, typically to store it in the dan tien, the middle balance point of the body located a couple inches below the navel, using the breath to do so. There are several variations of doing this but here are the basics.

In doing this exercise you'll want the tongue resting on the roof of the mouth with the mouth closed. Both the inhale and exhale are done through the nose. You'll also pull up on the perineum muscle, as covered in the breathing for strength section. Both of these are important for completing the circuit of the governing and central vessels, allowing the energy to flow and not leak.

Inhale, pulling the energy up the spine or governing channel, circling around the skull. Then exhale down the front center line of the body, the conception or central vessel. The starting and ending point is the dan tien. After the energy has reached here, you start the breath once again, completing the orbit over and over again.

The microcosmic orbit is used to aid in longevity, for mastering sexual energy, to enhance spirituality and much more. Once again, this is a very basic instruction of this technique. And if you want to go much further with it you'll want to consult with other texts and teachers such as the work of Mantak Chia.

Chakra Alignment Breathing

The following is a powerful drill I learned from one of my teachers, Dr. John La Tourrette. It helps balance all of the chakras and other energies in the body. This is a drill I tend to do each morning because it accomplishes a lot in a minimal amount of time.

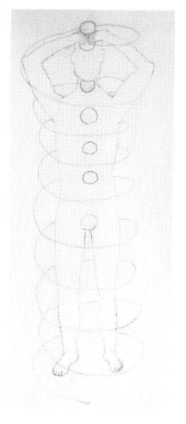

Think of a clockwise spiral of energy moving up your body. By that, I mean envision a clock laying on the ground with 12:00 being in front of you. Going clockwise from this appears to be the natural flow of the energy and to do it counter-clockwise does not feel right.

This spiral continues up the body, going through each chakra and ultimately coming out of the third eye. This is commonly thought of as the 6th chakra; however, certain people place the accurate flow of the chakras from the fifth at the throat, up to the seventh at the crown and then to the sixth at the third eye. This makes sense if you envision a cane or if you tilt your head back and think of tracking the spine up the back, to the top of the skull, and over to the front.

It is helpful to not only visualize the spiral of energy, feeling it moving throughout your body, but to trace the pattern with your arms. Now you want to imagine the spiral surrounding your entire body, but you can't trace it in the same way with your hands. The key is to feel the movement and energy flow.

Trace the spiral all the way up the body while inhaling. You will start near the feet while bent over and then come erect as you move up the body. Place the fingertips on the third eye while holding your breath at the top, your neck bent backward so your head faces up. Now, release the hands up and to the outside while you exhale. If you find yourself yawning during or after this exercise that is a good sign, as it is often a sign of the energy channels hooking up, or at least shifting to some degree.

Keep your body as relaxed as possible throughout this exercise. Any tension can constrict the flow of energy. Repeat the exercise three to five times. Note how you feel after doing it versus before. This can be a great thing to do a couple times throughout your day to help keep your energies flowing well.

Running Energy

While there are certainly going to be many forms of running energy, one of the simplest is breathing in, and then circulating the energy out of the hands as you breathe out. I personally like to inhale in the same manner as covered in the previous exercise with the clockwise spiral running up the body, the energy then coming out of the hands and the third eye at the same time.

Note that to do this effectively will take practice. But it's really not too difficult to do. And its effects can be felt not just by yourself but by another person who has some calibration skills.

There are multiple applications of this, from healing, to pretty much any of the other purposes of breathing we've covered here. This concept can be further explored in the *Quantum Touch* materials by Richard Gordon.

EFT Constricted Breathing Technique

EFT stands for Emotional Freedom Technique and is the most popular form of what is commonly called energy psychology or meridian tapping. At its basics, it involves saying phrases while tapping on meridian endpoints, pictured here, blending elements of Eastern and Western psychology. There is a lot of information on the subject out there, entire books cover this technique, so I won't go into all the details about how or why it works here. Suffice to say that in my experience it can be one of the most powerful and quickest ways of bringing about change.

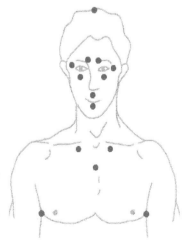

One of the techniques that is taught in EFT is known as the constricted breathing technique. Since it has to do with the breath it is worth sharing. This shows how the emotional or energetic component can have an effect on the physical. It is also because of this technique I came up with the *Instant Energy Exercise Enhancer*, as I found that if tapping could change the movement of breathing, it could change other movements as well.

This is also a great starting technique to use with EFT, as most often it gives people direct evidence in their own bodies showing them that it works.

To start, take a few deep breaths. This is to get the lungs warmed up. If you only took a deep breath once and measured against that, it could simply be from stretching the lungs a little further. Thus by taking a few deep breaths, we have already warmed and stretched the lungs out to a degree, thus the effects from the tapping are from the tapping, not that. After having done so, take a deep breath and note on a scale of 1 to 10 how deep your breathing is, with ten being the deepest breath you've even done, and one being not deep at all.

Then you begin tapping on the points, pictured here, while saying the setup and reminder phrases along the lines of "Even though my breathing feels a little constricted, I deeply love and accept myself," and "my breathing is constricted." If you're unfamiliar with the technique, I cover the basics of it in this series of articles I wrote for Breaking Muscle:

http://breakingmuscle.com/mind-body/is-eft-the-secret-to-enhanced-athletic-performance
http://breakingmuscle.com/mind-body/how-to-use-eft-to-overcome-challenges-in-the-gym

After you have gone through at least one complete round of tapping, take another deep breath and note if it has changed on your scale of 1 to 10 again. You may repeat several rounds and note further improvement.

Not everyone will feel the difference in breathing, though in my experience, the majority do. This can be a useful exercise to do before any other breathing exercises, which may further enhance the benefits you get, and possibly allow you to get them faster too. Try doing this before breath holds, and see if it can help you to go longer.

Holotropic Breathwork

The word holotropic means "moving towards wholeness." It is a process that was created by Dr. Stanislav Grof. Dr. Grof had been experimenting with psychedelic drugs like LSD for therapy, but when they were made illegal he turned to using the breath instead. He found that through breathing, you could induce altered states of consciousness that could be used for therapeutic purposes.

The basics of the process is to breathe deeper and faster than normal. In doing so, you typically breathe through the mouth to allow more air in and out faster. And there is no pause between inhaling and exhaling. This is done in a relaxed setting with music and for extended periods of time in which emotional release of stored traumas can occur for the aim of physical, energetic and emotional healing.

I have not personally done holotropic breathwork, but mention it for the sake of completeness. This technique is best done under the supervision of a certified holotropic breathwork practitioner. Important to note is that in doing some of the other forms of breathwork we have covered, which are similar to this, these same emotions or traumas may possibly arise.

Sample Routines

"Breath is spirit. The act of breathing is living." - *Author Unknown*

Many of the above techniques may be combined in a limitless variety of ways. I highly encourage you to experiment with doing so to find what works best for you.

Obviously, the strength, endurance and flexibility breathing exercises are best used when you're specifically working at exercises that do such a thing. So for the following discussion we'll keep those separate. What remains is the deep, lung capacity, relaxation, and energy breathing exercises.

Early in my physical training career, when I first got into breathing exercises, my routine looked something like the following.

1. Mighty Atom Exercise (10-20 reps)
2. Breathing with Arms Forward and Back (10-20 reps)
3. Breathing with Forward and Back Bending (10-20 reps)
4. Full Tidal Breathing (10-20 reps)
5. Abdominal Vacuum (5-10 reps)

This would often act as part of a warmup before any sort of workout. This is an excellent starting place for many people to begin.

More recently, each morning I've been starting my day off with a fairly simple routine. I offer this not to say you should do the exact same, but to give you examples of what I've done, so that you can gain ideas of how all we've covered can possibly be put together.

1. Abdominal Vacuum (3 reps)
2. Chakra Alignment Breathing (3 reps)
3. Breath Holds for Time (3 progressively longer holds, done with the Wim Hof Breathing or Hyperventilating in between. If I'm short on time, since this part takes much more than the rest, I'll do a single set or two of Exercise with Breath Holds, typically bodyweight squats.)

Then when I sit down to begin my meditative practice a short time later, I'll begin with Alternate Nostril Breathing. Sometimes I do this just in a regular relaxed breath, but other times I do it along with the Box Breathing or Centering Breath (4-4-4-4 or 6-2-7).

Alternatively, instead of breath holds, I'll engage in the Breath of Fire for a few minutes. You'll note that it is not always the exact same thing, but is constantly evolving.

While benefits can be gotten from a single deeper breath, if you're looking for longer last changes to how your breathing and your body operates, you'll want to spend at least ten minutes engaged in breathing exercises.

Besides having a breathing routine, recall that we talked about changing your habits of breathing from shallow, empty, and mouth breathing to deeper, fuller, and through the nose. So I wanted to offer some tips specifically on habit changes. First of all, a breathing routine as listed above will certainly be a helpful piece.

But in addition to that, you'll want to check on your breathing regularly, and do a couple conscious deep breathing exercises throughout your day. The easiest method, since what stops most people from doing something simple like this is just memory, and getting busy with other things, is to set a frequent alarm or timer. Most everyone has their mobile phone on them at all times, so put that technology to good use.

Set a timer every thirty minutes or every hour. When it beeps, check in with your breathing. Is it shallow or deep? Is it empty or full? Is it through the mouth or nose? Notice what you were doing. Then take a few deep breaths using any of the methods you'd like. Repeat the same thing the next time the timer goes off.

You can also build your deep breathing into other environmental triggers, besides an alarm going off. Perhaps every time you walk into a certain room, you'll take a deep breath or two. The important part is to build it into your day on a habitual level so that more healthful breathing becomes a natural part of who you are.

Your Air Environment

In this section of the book, we switch gears to talk not about how you breathe, but what you are breathing and the many things we can do to improve air quality.

It should go without saying that any type of deep breathing exercise will be better for you if you're breathing in good quality air. That being said, deep breathing in a polluted air environment like a city, is still better than not deep breathing at all. The only time you would want not to breathe is when there is something acutely poisonous around.

There are a variety of methods that we can use in order to improve our air quality. The first of which is mentioned by Burns above. The best time for a breathing routine is in the morning. The air is freshest outside at that time. Make use of it. That's not to say that if you can't do a breathing routine then, it's not worth doing. I'd say the other best time for deep breathing is anytime!

The following methods are especially important in our homes because that is where we spend most of our time.

Air is meant to circulate. And this is best done in a natural manner, rather than with air conditioning machines. The wind blows and air moves. So for the most part you should make use of this natural method. Besides being outside as often as you can, when you are indoors this means that the windows should be kept open when possible.

Screens can be used where bugs are a problem. If it is very cold in the area perhaps you can do it for just short amounts of time, like in the morning that we just discussed.

And even if you live in a city with less than best quality air, it is likely that keeping the windows open to circulate air, is better than that same poor quality air being stagnant.

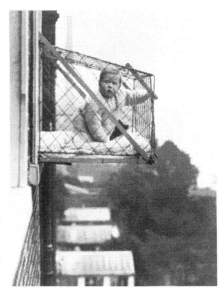

The best time and place to do this is in your bedroom while sleeping. Think about spending eight hours breathing the same air over and over again, especially at a point where your body is healing and repairing itself. It is much better to have fresh air during that time. If it's cold, that's not so much a problem as you can simply get under more blankets.

My favorite example of taking this to an extreme is this picture which I found in one of Bernarr MacFadden's books. Now I wouldn't recommend doing this, what I like to call the baby cage, but it also goes to show you the importance placed on fresh air and sunlight.

Humidity

The humidity of the air, which is the quantity of water in it, may be another important factor. For some people a dryer climate will help, typically because they're too damp internally. For others the opposite will be the case.

A humidifier can be used indoors to make dry air more humid. Different humidifiers will keep the moisture cool, while other ones can warm it up. These can also be used to aid in constitutional balancing.

There is one possible drawback. You will want to be careful in using these as harmful molds and bacteria tend to like humid conditions, and you don't want to trigger their growth inside your home. I personally don't feel the need to use a humidifier in my area, so I can't make a good recommendation on what you might get if you feel you need one.

Forest Bathing

Recent research has come out showing the benefits of forest bathing, or Shinrin-yoku, as it is known in Japanese and Mandarin. These include reductions in stress, anger, anxiety, depression and better sleep. Hormonal changes have been noted in cortisol and adiponectin as well.[7]

One of the reasons for this is the quality of the air. In a forest surrounded by trees you'll be breathing in phytoncides or wood essential oils. Not only do these provide the benefits above, but many are antibacterial as well. I've heard it said that certain forests are actually cleaner than hospitals because of these compounds.

There is a reason I love living close to the forest. Of course, the air quality is only one of the many benefits. Even if you live in the city, you would want to find time to get out to nature when you can. I doubt that forests are the only beneficial types of nature either.

Even a park inside a dense city is bound to have some of these benefits. I'd bet that various bodies of water would bring about many of the same benefits too. If you can't access a forest regularly, this effect may be mimicked at least in part through the following method indoors.

Diffusers and Nebulizers

Besides the humidifier that is mentioned above, there are other devices that would help improve your air quality indoors that I think would be useful for all people.

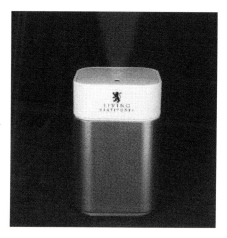

A diffuser is a device that allows you to evaporate any liquid through heat. Thus, you can use tree essential oils to get a similar forest bathing effect. You can also use any variety of other herbal essential oils for their effects too.

A nebulizer is similar in effects but it nebulizes the liquid, which is a process that breaks down essential oils into very small particles, which then are spread throughout the air. It requires a high velocity pressurized air stream. Nebulization may be the better option because it keeps the molecules intact, without using heat, but separated so that they can more easily get into the lungs and not filtered out.

The Living Beatitudes Nebulizer is highly recommended. I just picked up this unit and keep it running in my office while I do work. In fact, it's running right now nearby while I write this with a pine essential oil.

http://legendarystrength.com/go/nebulizer/

Air Purifier

As the name implies these devices help to clear the air of many particles that aren't the best for your health. One of the things you'll want to look for in this device is a HEPA filter, which stands for high efficiency particulate air. To be classified as a HEPA filter the device must meet particular standards of removing 99.97% of airborne particles 0.3 micrometers in diameter.

Sometimes UV light is also built in. UV light is capable of destroying airborne bacteria, viruses, fungi and more. However, there is debate as to whether the UV units on many of these filters will contact enough of the air to make much of a difference in this regard.

Some units also produce ozone. And while ozone can be used in smart ways, having it emitted by an air purifier may not be the best option. California has banned the sale of any unit emitting more than 50 parts per billion of ozone from being sold.

The size of the unit is a large part of how much area it can cover. Smaller units work for small rooms, while you might need something bigger if it's the only one in your house. A good practice, if you only have one air purifier, is to move it around from room to room over time.

Upon searching, I came across the fact that an airborne-particle physicist, using $100000 of equipment, set out to test the different air purifiers on the market. The Coway AP-1512HH Mighty Air Purifier appears to be the winner for the most effective and at the same time cost effective. It beat out units twice its size and twice the price.

http://legendarystrength.com/go/airpurifier/

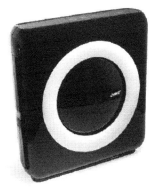

Plants

Although technology can be useful, let's not skip the most important detail. Plants create oxygen. They basically breathe the inverse of us, taking in our carbon dioxide and breathing out oxygen. When it comes to breath, we live symbiotically with them.

And here's the good news. Plants do even more for the air than just produce oxygen. They can also clean the area of various sorts of chemicals that our homes unfortunately are full of, from flame retardants on furniture and mattresses, to many cleaning supplies and much more.

NASA conducted a study back in 1989 to find ways to clean the air in space stations[8]. It was found that certain plants cleaned specific chemicals like benzene, formaldehyde, toluene, and ammonia. The chart on the following page, copied from Wikipedia, showcases these findings.

After hearing about this, I ran down to my local gardening store and picked up several of these plants. Just a couple feet away from my desk as I write this is a large snake plant, also known as "Mother-in-Law's Tongue". Not only do these clean the air very well, but they require very little watering, making it a great plant even for those with the brownest of thumbs.

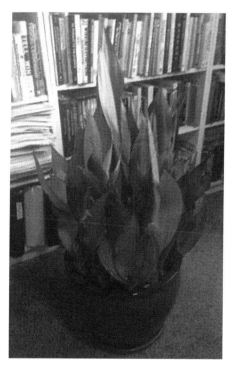

The truth is that pretty much all plants will be beneficial, though when it comes to cleaning the air, what is listed on the next page is probably a good place to start. I would also argue that living among plants will do more for us than produce oxygen and clean the air, but that's another topic for another time.

So if we can't get to the forest every day for a dose of forest bathing, we can bring some of the forest to us in the form of plants and their essential oils.

The common name of the plants are listed in the chart below. A 'yes' indicates that plant helps to remove that chemical from the air.

Plant	Benzene	Formaldehyde	Trichloroethylene	Xylene/Toulene	Ammonia
Dwarf date palm	No	Yes	No	Yes	No
Areca palm	No	Yes	No	Yes	No
Boston fern	No	Yes	No	Yes	No
Kimberly queen fern	No	Yes	No	Yes	No
English ivy	Yes	Yes	Yes	Yes	No
Lilyturf	No	Yes	No	Yes	Yes
Spider plant	No	Yes	No	Yes	No
Devil's ivy	Yes	Yes	No	Yes	No
Peace lily	Yes	Yes	Yes	Yes	Yes
Flamingo lily	No	Yes	No	Yes	Yes
Chinese evergreen	Yes	Yes	No	No	No
Bamboo palm	No	Yes	No	Yes	No
Broadleaf lady palm	No	Yes	No	Yes	Yes
Variegated snake plant	Yes	Yes	Yes	Yes	No
Heartleaf philodendron	No	Yes	No	No	No
Selloum philodendron	No	Yes	No	No	No
Elephant ear philodendron	No	Yes	No	No	No
Red-edged dracaena	Yes	Yes	Yes	Yes	No
Cornstalk dracaena	Yes	Yes	Yes	No	No
Weeping Fig	No	Yes	No	Yes	No
Barberton daisy	Yes	Yes	Yes	No	No
Florist's chrysanthemum	Yes	Yes	Yes	Yes	Yes
Rubber plant	No	Yes	No	No	No
Dendrobium orchids	No	No	No	Yes	No
Dumb canes	No	No	No	Yes	No
King of hearts	No	No	No	Yes	No
Moth orchids	No	No	No	Yes	No

Measuring Indoor Air Quality

I believe that most of these steps are useful to do no matter where you are. But for those that are looking for more data about their air quality before they begin there are a couple options.

It looks like the market is starting to see a number of items that regularly test for things like VOC's and particle matter in the air. Here are websites for two such devices:

- http://getbirdi.com/
- http://foobot.io/

The one thing these devices do not test is for mold specifically. There may be some other testing options that could look at this on an airborne level.

Respiratory Herbs

"If a heavy charge was made for the three foregoing, the "big three" of nature cure – fresh air, pure water and walking exercise – what a rush there would be for them!" – Thomas Inch

This book is not meant to be a guide to clearing colds and flus. That being said, since we've talked about the respiratory tract, it would be good to mention a few things. Generally, simple illnesses like the cold or flus occur because viruses get into our system. As such, the infection typically begins in the upper respiratory tract and many symptoms occur in the same area.

But by supporting the area, we can often change the ecology of these areas and thus help our immune system to fight off these pathogens.

In cases where the lungs just seem weak overall, one of the best herbs for its recovery is Cordyceps. This isn't just for weakness, but for its tonic effects too. Many people notice their endurance increases with regular use of cordyceps, myself included. In fact, this fascinating fungus is what really got me hooked on the herbal world, as I noticed a distinct benefit in my workouts when using it. Although I was originally using the *Cordyceps sinensis*, I've since found that, at least with this supply, the *Cordyceps militaris* works ever better. Find out more and get some at https://lostempireherbs.com/product/cordyceps/

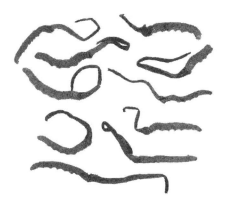

In Chinese medicine, there are many other great herbs that help support the lungs in different ways. These include asparagus root and goji berries for moistening the lungs, codonopsis for tonic effects, licorice for clearing, ma huang or ephedra for stimulation, as well as many others.

In the West, there are different herbs available. In cases of allergies, beyond changes in diet which can lower the overall allergic load and are often at the root of chronic allergy problems, there are a few herbs that may assist. Histamine can be cleared using St. John's wort, rosemary, nettle leaf and licorice.

Using a diffuser or nebulizer of essential oils of peppermint, rosemary, thyme, sage, eucalyptus or chamomile may be the best way for internal topical delivery of the lungs and respiratory tract to assist in these cases. More standard delivery means of teas, powders, tinctures and pills will also work but when in doubt, go directly to the area affected.

In cases of asthma or fits of coughing, herbs that are antispasmodic include lobelia and thyme. Coltsfoot is also useful, and was a favorite of Native Americans.

Expectoration is an action which helps the body to remove infected mucus from the lungs and body. This herbal action should be used when there is dampness in the lungs, as opposed to say a dry cough. Several of these include osha, lomatium, oregano, lobelia, mullein, wild cherry and pleurisy root.

In those dry cases, a demulcent action can help. Demulcent herbs include marshmallow, slippery elm, comfrey, licorice, plantain and mullein. You'll notice that mullein was in both damp and dry lists, indicating its dual-direction activity.

A decongestant action can be found with horseradish, garlic, eyebright, elderflower and more.

Many people first feel a cold coming on by a sore throat. In cases like this, you can do a simple gargle of sage, chamomile, lemon, honey and salt. Make a tea of the first two then add the last three. Gargle with this several times throughout the day.

There is a whole lot more that can be covered in this area; again, entire books are written on this one topic, but hopefully by just seeing the different things herbs can do, you may reach for these the next time you need them. You want to support the body in clearing the infection rather than suppressing it. Cough medicine, and most of our pharmaceutical drugs, typically suppress the symptoms, and thus lengthens the illness as the body can't clear it out.

Using some of these herbs, as well as others, on a semi-regular basis can help you to keep your health in top condition and thus avoid things like the common cold. If your immune system is working close to optimal, and your various points of entry for germs in the body are not in a condition to support their attachment and reproduction, then avoiding illness is easy enough to accomplish. This is true even if you are surrounded by sick people.

Further, by having a healthy respiratory system, both the upper and lower portions of it, it will make all the breathing exercises both easier to do and more effective. Each side will support the other.

Upgrade Your Breathing Action Checklist

"The wisest one-word sentence? Breathe." - Terri Guillemets

This checklist is a bit smaller than others in the Upgrade Your Health series. The reason for this is that most of the information covered here was about different possibilities of breathing exercises. No one should do them all, at least at any one time.

The important thing is to use the right types for you in the right applications, as well as build a routine that can serve you over time, even though it may be continually evolving. Most of the things listed below are best done ongoing and long-term.

☐ Make Breathing Deeply and Fully a Habit

☐ Make Nasal Breathing a Habit

☐ Develop a Daily Breathing Exercise Routine

☐ Work up to a 3+ Minute Breath Hold

☐ Keep Your Windows Open (as much as possible)

☐ Surround Your Indoors with Oxygen Producing and Toxin Eliminating Plants

☐ Get an Air Purifier

☐ Get a Nebulizer

☐ Regularly Spend Time in Nature

☐ Use the Tonic Herb Cordyceps

☐ Have Other Herbs on Hand that are Useful for Different Respiratory Issues

Conclusion

"Breath is the bridge which connects life to consciousness,
which unites your body to your thoughts."
- Thích Nhất Hạnh

We have covered a lot of breathing information in this book. Far more than you're likely to put into action in your life, at least at one time. But even if you use just a single breathing exercise, and do one thing to improve the quality of your air environment, this book has achieved its aim to help you upgrade your breathing.

Of course, you can do much more than a single exercise. The best option would be to experiment with a number of different exercises, and develop your own breathing routine that you practice every single day. As there are lots of things you can do, over time this routine should evolve. What you need to start out with in breathing exercises will not be the same as what you will need a year later after practicing them.

For those reasons, think of this book as a reference manual that can and should be returned to over time. As you read this, I'm sure a few exercises stood out to you and piqued your interest. Start with those. But when you return to this guide later, new exercises will stand out in a new way because you and your breathing have changed. And then you should begin to work with those.

While this is probably one of the most comprehensive guides on breathing out there, there is no way that it could cover every single method or application of breathing. Many of the ideas were only touched upon, when entire books could be, and have been, written about a single one of them. Still I believe with what has been covered, you will have a greater grasp of what can be done with your breath then the majority of people alive.

But this is only as useful as what you do with it. Without a breathing practice, these words will do nothing for you. So, I encourage you right now to stop reading, as it's the end of this book anyway, and choose one exercise to do some breathing practice right now.

Be sure to let me know how these practices work out for you. I love hearing feedback so send an email my way at logan@legendarystrength.com.

Recommended Reading

Breathology, Stig Åvall Severinsen
http://legendarystrength.com/go/breathology

Evolve Your Breathing, Jon Haas
http://legendarystrength.com/go/evolveyourbreathing/

The Spiritual Journey of Joseph L. Greenstein, Ed Spielman
http://legendarystrength.com/go/mightyatom/

Maxalding, Monte Saldo
http://legendarystrength.com/go/maxalding/

Muscle Control, Maxick
http://legendarystrength.com/go/musclecontrol/

The Key to Might and Muscle, George Jowett
http://legendarystrength.com/go/jowett/

Lessons in Wrestling and Physical Culture, Martin Farmer Burns
http://legendarystrength.com/go/farmerburns/

My Breathing System, J.P. Mueller
http://legendarystrength.com/go/mueller/

The Naked Warrior, Pavel Tsatsouline
http://legendarystrength.com/nakedwarrior/

Awareness through Movement, Moshe Feldenkrais
http://legendarystrength.com/go/feldenkrais/

Awaken Healing Energy through the Tao, Mantak Chia
http://legendarystrength.com/go/tao/

Quantum Touch, Richard Gordon
http://legendarystrength.com/go/quantumtouch/

Recommended Watching

The Wim Hof Method Online Program, Wim Hof
http://legendarystrength.com/go/wimhof/

Be Breathed DVD, Scott Sonnon
http://legendarystrength.com/go/bebreathed/

Master Muscle Control, Logan Christopher
http://musclecontrolexercises.com/

Scientific References

1. Kannel, W., Seidman, J., Fercho, W., & Castelli, W. (1974). Vital Capacity and Congestive Heart Failure: The Framingham Study. *Circulation,* 1160-1166. http://circ.ahajournals.org/content/49/6/1160.full.pdf

2. Sharma, G., & Goodwin, J. Effect of aging on respiratory system physiology and immunology. *Clinical Interventions in Aging,* 253-260. http://www.ncbi.nlm.nih.gov/pmc/articles/PMC2695176/

3. Lundberg, J., Settergren, G., Gelinder, S., Lundberg, J., Alving, K., & Weitzberg, E. (n.d.). Inhalation of nasally derived nitric oxide modulates pulmonary function in humans. *Acta Physiol Scand Acta Physiologica Scandinavica,* 343-347. http://www.ncbi.nlm.nih.gov/pubmed/8971255

4. Kox, M., Eijk, L., Zwaag, J., Wildenberg, J., Sweep, F., Hoeven, J., & Pickkers, P. (2014). Voluntary activation of the sympathetic nervous system and attenuation of the innate immune response in humans. *Proceedings of the National Academy of Sciences,* 7379-7384. http://www.icemanwimhof.com/files/pnas.pdf

5. Baković, D., Valic, Z., Eterović, D., Vuković, I., Obad, A., Marinović-Terzić, I., & Dujić, Z. (2003). Spleen volume and blood flow response to repeated breath-hold apneas. *Journal of Applied Physiology J Appl Physiol,* 1460-1466. http://www.ncbi.nlm.nih.gov/pubmed/12819225

6. Donaldson, VW (2000). A clinical study of visualization on depressed white blood cell count in medical patients. *Applied Psychophysiology and Biofeedback,* 117-128 http://www.ncbi.nlm.nih.gov/pubmed/10932336

7. Tsunetsugu, Y., Park, B., & Miyazaki, Y. (2009). Trends in research related to "Shinrin-yoku" (taking in the forest atmosphere or forest bathing) in Japan. *Environmental Health and Preventive Medicine Environ Health Prev Med,* 27-37. http://www.ncbi.nlm.nih.gov/pubmed/19585091

8. BC Wolverton, WL Douglas, K Bounds (July 1989). A study of interior landscape plants for indoor air pollution abatement (Report). NASA. NASA-TM-108061. http://ntrs.nasa.gov/archive/nasa/casi.ntrs.nasa.gov/19930073077.pdf

About the Author

Born without genetic gifts, a weak and scrawny Logan Christopher sought out the best training information in his pursuit of super strength, mind power and radiant health. Nowadays, he's known for his famous feats of pulling an 8,800 lb. firetruck by his hair, juggling flaming kettlebells, and supporting half a ton in the wrestler's bridge. Called the "Physical Culture Renaissance Man" his typical workouts might include backflips, freestanding handstand pushups, tearing phonebooks in half, bending steel, deadlifting a heavy barbell, or lifting rocks overhead.

Far from being all brawn and no brain Logan has sought optimal performance with mental training and sports psychology which he has explored in depth, becoming an NLP Trainer, certified hypnotist, EFT practitioner and more. That's also how he got started in the field of health and nutrition which inevitably led to Chinese, Ayurvedic and Western herbalism.

His personal philosophy is to bring together the best movement skill, health information, and mental training to achieve peak performance. He is the author of many books and video programs to help people increase their strength, skills, health and mental performance. Discover how you too can become super strong, both mentally and physically, at www.LegendaryStrength.com and find the superior herbs to support all aspects of your performance at www.SuperManHerbs.com.

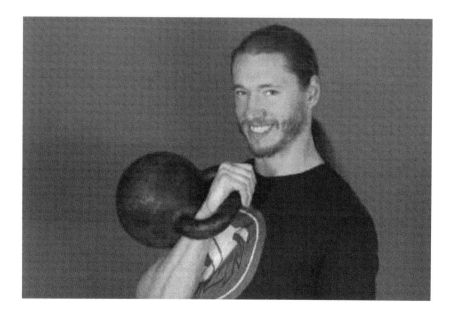

Other Books in the Upgrade Your Health Series:

Upgrade Your Testosterone http://legendarystrength.com/testosterone/

Upgrade Your Growth Hormone http://legendarystrength.com/growth-hormone/

Upgrade Your Water http://legendarystrength.com/upgrade-your-water/

Upgrade Your Sleep http://legendarystrength.com/upgrade-your-sleep/

Upgrade Your Fat http://legendarystrength.com/upgrade-your-fat/

Upgrade Your Vitamins http://legendarystrength.com/upgrade-your-vitamins/

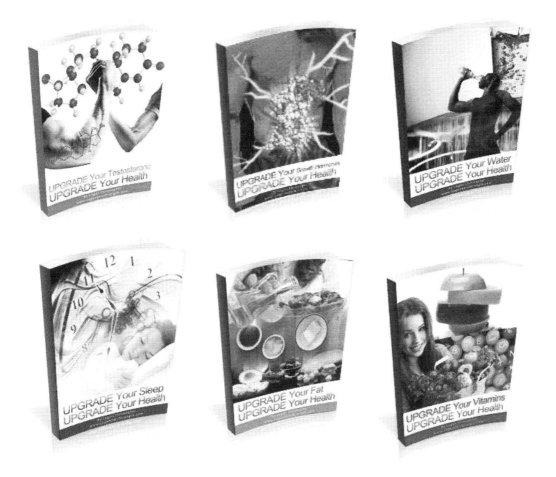

**For a full up-to-date of titles in the Upgrade Your Health Series plus more books
and videos from Logan Christopher go to:
http://www.LegendaryStrength.com/books-videos/**

"Get Stronger... Move Better... Become Healthier... Unleash Your Mind Power... Every Single Month"

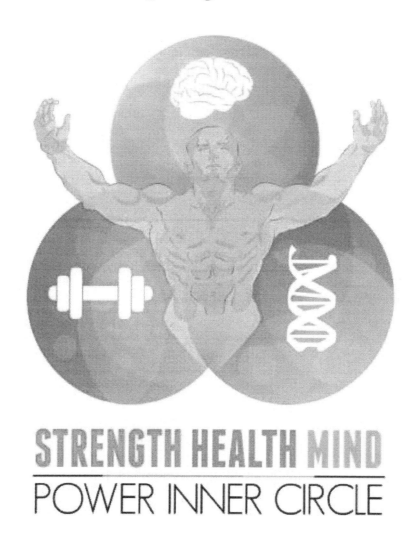

STRENGTH HEALTH MIND
POWER INNER CIRCLE

- Monthly Newsletter on Achieving Peak Health & Performance
- Access to Coaching from Logan Christopher
- Private Community of Members
- Free Bonuses and Videos
- And Much More

Go to www.StrengthHealthMindPower.com

Made in the USA
Middletown, DE
23 May 2021

39953300R00044